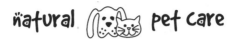
natural pet care

Allergies

D0631196

BY LISA S. NEWMAN, N.D., Ph.D

Foreword by Deborah C. Mallu, D.V.M., C.V.A.

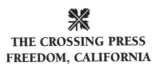

THE CROSSING PRESS
FREEDOM, CALIFORNIA

Copyright © 1999 by Lisa S. Newman
Cover photographs by Quarto, Inc. for Artville
Printed in the U.S.A.

*No part of this publication may be reproduced or transmitted in any form
or by any means, electric or mechanical, including photocopy, recording,
or any information storage and retrieval system now known or to be in-
vented, without permission in writing from the publisher, except by a
reviewer who wishes to quote brief passages in connection with a review
written for inclusion in a magazine, newspaper, or broadcast. Contact
The Crossing Press, Inc., P.O. Box 1048, Freedom, CA 95019.*

All rights reserved.

For information on bulk purchases or group discounts for this and other
Crossing Press titles, please contact our Special Sales Manager at
800/777-1048. Visit our web site: **www.crossingpress.com**

Cautionary Note: The nutritional information, recipes, and instructions contained within this book are in no way intended as a substitute
for medical counseling. Please do not attempt self-treatment of a medical problem without consulting a qualified health practitioner.

The author and The Crossing Press expressly disclaim any and all lia-
bility for any claims, damages, losses, judgments, expenses, costs, and
liabilities of any kind or injuries resulting from any products offered
in this book by participating companies and their employees or agents.
Nor does the inclusion of any resource group or company listed within this book constitute an endorsement or guarantee of quality by the
author or The Crossing Press.

Library of Congress Cataloging-in-Publication Data
Newman, Lisa S.
    Allergies / by Lisa S. Newman.
        p. cm. -- (The Crossing Press pocket series. Natural pet care.)
    ISBN 1-58091-002-5 (pbk.)
    1. Allergy in dogs. 2. Allergy in cats. 3. Dogs--Diseases-
-Alternative treatment. 4. Cats--Diseases--Alternative treatment.
5. Holistic veterinary medicine. I. Title. II. Series.
SF992.A44N48   1999
636.7'089697--dc21
                                              99-37387
                                                  CIP

Contents

Foreword

It is with great pleasure that I introduce Lisa Newman's remarkable series. She has dedicated her life to helping you care for your animal companions—we can all benefit from her years of experience.

We are living in a time of great change, especially in the realm of health care. As a practicing veterinarian for more than two decades, I have witnessed both myself and my clients begin to seek less invasive, more natural methods for healing our dogs and cats. Once we understood that all beings are interconnected on this planet, we became aware that our thoughts, emotions, and family dynamics played an important role in the health of our animal companions. We began to realize the importance of forming a team first with the members of our animal family, aided by other healing professionals including natural health counselors and animal communicators.

Over the years I have heard people say, "I didn't know you could use that natural remedy or treatment on animals." Feel confident that you can help your animal companions where the healing is best—in your loving home. Our animals nurture us by giving us unconditional love. In turn, we can nurture them with fresh, live food and supplements, so that they can live a long and healthy life. Lisa Newman will show you the way so that you can be empowered as a healer.

Deborah C. Mallu, D.V.M., C.V.A.

What Is a Reaction?

An allergy is the body's intense reaction to a substance called an allergen. An allergen can be inhaled through the lungs, ingested through the mouth, or absorbed by the skin. Often, when these substances are eliminated, symptoms do seem to decrease. Pets exhibit their distress by scratching and/or biting their bodies. Other symptoms include digestive upsets, body odor, poor coats, and difficult breathing.

Many pet owners feel frustrated because though they treat their pet's allergies year after year, there is little long-term relief. As time passes, the allergic symptoms generally get worse. Owners will try almost anything: eliminate the supposed substance that is causing the trouble; search for the next medication or dietary change. Usually with each passing season the animal becomes weaker, the medications become less effective, and the diets prove to be a waste of money. It's an endless, desperate battle.

Allergies are a common sign that the body is not being cared for as nature intended. As time passes, the pet's immune system gets weaker, placing additional stress on the body's other systems, until the whole body breaks down. It is, therefore, not unusual to see the more serious diseases such as cancer in older animals with a history of allergies.

It is my belief that many allergies simply indicate an imbalance in the immune system, not a true sensitivity to one substance. I have found fewer than twenty percent of animals with suspected allergies have been correctly diagnosed, and the remaining eighty percent are suffering from a depressed immune system and an unbalanced diet.

Allopathic veterinary medicine, our country's standard medical care, does not yet fully understand how the immune system works. It lumps symptoms under a general diagnosis and then tries to suppress them, rather than treating the body as a whole. Here's a short scenario on how the body works: A pet's body is constantly being confronted with dangerous substances, in the environment (for example, pesticides in the house), or in commercial pet food that contains animal by-products, rancid animal fat, and grain by-products (all common pet food ingredients). Waste products build up in the body, and the whole digestive system suffers. The skin, the body's largest eliminatory organ, then tries to release these waste products. This results in pimples, rashes, and hot spots. Urea, a waste product of protein digestion, promotes a gout-like condition, which can cause the animal to start chewing and scratching itself.

Steroids, commonly used to reduce inflammation, will temporarily reduce the allergic symptoms by reducing the reaction to a toxin, but will not tackle the underlying problem of a depressed immune system. Though the symptoms appear to be reduced, the pet will not get better in the long run, and most animals probably will get worse.

To strengthen the immune system, it is necessary to cleanse the body of toxins. Supplements and homeopathic or herbal remedies will ensure that the fundamental imbalance is corrected. Feeding your pets at least twice a day and sometimes more if needed will help to keep their blood sugar stable and to keep the hormonal system balanced. It is important to provide proper grooming and an emotionally stable environment. You will find that this regimen will foster a strong immune system and the allergies will disappear.

The best defense for an allergic pet is a strong offense. The first step is to get a proper diagnosis from your veterinarian to ensure that you are not dealing with a serious illness. Whatever the problem, serious or minor, there are many natural protocols you can successfully follow.

Allergies as Symptoms

Inbreeding, and excessive genetic manipulation of the more popular breeds, has minimized our animals' natural curative abilities, leaving them very susceptible to allergies. Years of vaccinations, chemical baths, flea and tick potions, dips and sprays, medications, and most importantly, poor-quality ingredients, artificial colors, preservatives, and by-products found in most pet foods and treats, all take their toll.

It is important to distinguish a true allergy from a depressed immune system. Although the holistic protocol, the method of stimulating the body, is very similar in both cases, by defining allergies and understanding the relationship between an allergen and the body's reaction to it, you will be better prepared to address your own animal's individual needs and effectively reverse their condition, regardless of the cause.

The diagnosis of allergies has become too inclusive. Many conditions—poor skin and coat conditions, digestive upsets, respiratory problems, arthritis, and poor immune function—are often explained as allergic reactions. Some hypersensitivity reactions are true pathological processes that are triggered by the interaction of specific allergens: The resulting symptom is caused by a true allergy.

Holistically, I see all "allergies" as strictly symptoms, rather than conditions. Even true allergies, whether the allergen is ingested, inhaled, or a chemical irritation, are typically just a form of hypersensitivity reaction. A specific allergic reaction is a symptom: Its underlying cause is rarely from the allergens themselves. Due to this difficulty of distinguishing between symptoms and causes, making a causative diagnosis and implementing a successful treatment protocol can be difficult.

Therapies that focus only on the removal of the allergen or the suppression of the allergic response, rather than addressing the root cause, will give symptomatic relief at best. At worst, they will cause chronic, more frequent cycling of the symptoms—which places enormous burdens on the vital organs. This will happen even if the therapy you choose is a holistic one.

You must look beyond the symptoms or sensitivities. Certainly, I do not advocate allowing an animal to suffer from an oozing hot spot without addressing it. But, looking deeper, for the *cause* of the irritation, and *addressing that imbalance* will be more effective. It will dry up the hot spot faster, and may prevent it from re-occurring.

There are three most commonly diagnosed allergy groups. You may be able to match your pet to one of these, or you may have already received a similar diagnosis. If you explore more deeply, you may find that the underlying cause is not a simple allergen. This deeper exploration may help you address your pet's symptoms more successfully, relieving them or reversing the sensitivity completely.

DEFINING ALLERGIES

There are three types of allergic irritants. The first are those that are inhaled by pets. Pets who have only airborne-related allergies, and whose symptoms are largely seasonal, are often diagnosed with sensitivities to inhaled allergens. Symptoms associated with inhaled allergens can include:

- general redness and itching of the skin with rashes or pustules (especially around the face, belly, and feet)
- hair loss and poor coat condition (brittle with dandruff or greasy)
- fur picking and poor coat growth or sheen
- ear or eye infections

- upper respiratory problems including asthma, excessive salivation, or nasal discharge
- irritability and a nervous nature, including restlessness at night with endless licking, biting, picking, and scratching

Inhaled allergies are most often referred to as *airborne-related* symptoms. These are caused by pollen, dander, or dust. Sources can vary from flowering trees and grasses, to your pet's own coat, to household dust. This can be the most frustrating allergy to deal with, because all too often it is virtually impossible to completely eliminate the source. If an allopathic treatment is adopted, animals seem to develop a tolerance to prescribed or over-the-counter antihistamines fairly quickly. Allergy shots, the most popular treatment for airborne allergies, often become less effective each season, leaving both owner and pet frustrated.

A holistic approach may prove successful for animals in this category. Elimination of the source of the allergic response is almost impossible because it will be extremely difficult to trace, and the traditional allopathic approach often results in an overall decline of health. There is a solution: Addressing the underlying imbalance of the immune system holistically quickly reverses most symptoms and often completely eliminates the sensitivity to these allergens.

While symptom suppression alone can be successfully accomplished through natural methods, a *complete* holistic protocol of detoxification and nutritional and herbal supplementation is best. This protocol will stimulate the immune system, and lead to a more rapid and possibly more thorough reversal of the allergy condition or sensitivities.

The second type of allergy is an allergy caused by ingestion of foods or chemicals. Pets who have predominantly ingested-related allergies are not affected by environmental or chemical allergens, such as pollen or dips, or by changes in the season. Ingested allergens can include individual foods and treats, and also by-products and chemicals in foods, such as preservatives and artificial flavors. These pets most often suffer from:

- gastric upset including bloating (the number one food-related acute cause of death in dogs)
- gas, diarrhea and/or constipation, irritable bowel syndrome
- vomiting, hair balls
- ear and eye discharges and irritation
- skin and coat problems (including odor, hot spots, redness, and itching)
- general loss of vitality
- joint inflammation, arthritic pain
- organ failure
- excessive emotional/behavioral traits such as shyness, nervousness, or fear-aggression.

Ingested allergies, more commonly known as *food allergies*, are, in my opinion, the most misdiagnosed of allergic conditions; chemical-based allergies are a close second. There are over thirty different commercial and prescription "allergy relief" diets, yet our pets are still suffering from diarrhea, constipation, irritable bowel syndrome, gas, and vomiting. Despite this plethora of allergy-relief diets, the symptoms continue because the true problem is the poor quality of the ingredients in our pets' food and the body's inability to digest and assimilate them.

Beef was one of the first ingredients targeted by veterinarians as a prime allergen. Many pets who previously tested positive for a beef sensitivity are now eating high-quality beef regularly with no symptoms. Addressing food-related allergies holistically often results in a complete reversal of the symptoms.

The third type of allergy is caused by chemical irritation. Chemically irritated pets have a reaction to certain substances in their environment, including carpeting, shampoos, cigarette smoke, household cleaning products, vaccinations, pesticides, and even their own drinking water, beds, or collars. Chemical irritants can be produced by the body itself, as in the case of hormones. Or there may be insufficient chemical output from the endocrine system, as in the case of cortisol deficiency. Stress on other glands, such as the thyroid or pituitary, may also result from or contribute to allergies and the general imbalances associated with them. There is a wide range of symptoms to chemical irritants:

- ear and eye discharges and irritation
- gastric upset including bloating, as chemicals interfere with digestion and elimination, causing waste to back up in the bowel
- gas, diarrhea and/or constipation, irritable bowel syndrome
- vomiting, hair balls trapped in backed-up waste
- skin problems, including dandruff, hot spots, pimples, redness, and itching
- poor coat condition, including dry or greasy fur, coat loss, fur picking
- general loss of vitality
- joint inflammation, muscular and arthritic pain
- organ failure from chronic symptoms such as F.U.S. (Feline Urological Syndrome), cystitis, diabetes, and even poor elimination
- excessive emotional/behavioral traits such as complete isolation, nervousness, fearfulness, or aggression
- seizures
- cataracts
- diabetes
- cancer, especially fatty skin tumors, sarcomas, and leukemia
- loss of reproductive capabilities
- general immune system dysfunction

Chemically based allergies, also known as *environmental allergies*, are surprisingly common. Pets respond to their environment similar to the way we do, reacting to chemicals polluting their bodies. In some instances, our pets are exposed to far more chemicals than we ever are. Cats and dogs typically eat up to one-third their body weight in chemical preservatives each year, and are completely doused in chemical pesticides, which are then left on to be absorbed through the skin. When was the last time you took a bath in a lethal pesticide or wore a pesticide-laced collar daily?

Many pets spend a lot of time in direct contact with carpeting, floors, and outdoor landscapes that have been heavily treated with cleaning solutions, herbicides, and pesticides. This repeated exposure makes them more likely to develop sensitivities to these chemicals. Pets may spend their day outside breathing car exhaust, and their night inside, exposed to second-hand smoke. Even drinking water may be a culprit if it contains heavy metals, chemicals, bacteria, and amoebas. If you are not willing to drink your own tap water, then please do not give it to your animals.

Many pets may also suffer from multiple allergies, which cross between the three major categories. Multiple-allergy symptoms and the resulting decline of health can be overwhelming. Traditionally, the allopathic approach has been to treat the various symptoms with a variety of drugs that may successfully suppress the symptom and temporarily alleviate suffering. But once medication is stopped, symptoms commonly recur and often worsen with each recurrence, even though the original cause (such as a carpet) has been removed.

It is impossible to affect one aspect of the body without affecting the rest. Chronic drug use may result in organ failure. Death can result from an ongoing assault on the body and the immune system. Too often, a pet is euthanized to end its suffering after drugs can no longer suppress the symptoms.

I do not advocate allowing an animal to suffer unnecessarily. I recommend using a medication prescribed by your veterinarian in the event of a *life-threatening* imbalance, infection, or injury. However, I do strongly urge that you change your pet's diet and improve its digestion and environment to strengthen its body first. Drugs should be seen as a last resort, warranted only in an emergency, as in the case of anaphylactic shock, adrenal malfunction, or a life-threatening staphylococcal infection. Consult with a veterinarian you trust, and weigh the pros and cons of various treatments.

Assessing Allergies

To assess of the nature of your pet's allergic response and its severity, you must incorporate information that includes:

- how acute (immediate) or chronic (long-term) the onset of symptoms are
- the time (i.e., after meals or early morning) or season in which it is most aggravated
- determining exposure to allergens in the diet or environment
- clinical tests

Skin tests and blood tests are used to confirm that the agents involved in allergies are present through the detection of eosinophils, specific antibody levels, WBC (white blood cell) counts, and histamines released.

When the veterinarian finds that skin testing is contraindicated because of extreme dermatitis, the RAST (radioallergosorbent test) is performed. In this test, allergens are mixed with a sample of the animal's blood and specific antibodies (and therefore the extent of the allergy) are determined. Although the results of these medical tests cannot be disputed, the veterinarian's response to these results and the recommended course of treatment, whether allopathic or holistic, can differ greatly.

The allopathic veterinary practitioner will focus on the diagnosis of "allergies" and will seek to suppress symptoms through drugs (antihistamines, antibiotics, steroids for inflammation and immune stimulation). Based on test results, the veterinarian will attempt to identify the specific allergens responsible, so that they may be avoided. But all too often, shortly after the termination of medication, there is a full return of symptoms.

The holistic practitioner, on the other hand, will use these tests as confirmation of an underlying imbalance.

Initially, certain ingredients which have tested positive as an allergen may be avoided, and certain symptoms may be suppressed (preferably naturally). Emphasis is placed on stimulating the body's defense mechanisms (immune system) into reversing the condition, thereby eliminating the symptoms altogether. In a large percentage of animals, holistic animal care often allows the reintroduction of the very ingredients previously known to have triggered an allergy response.

ALLERGIES, SENSITIVITIES, OR TOXICITY?

Let us now explore and evaluate what a true allergy is, and determine how often sensitivities or even toxicity are the true culprits behind that so-called "allergic" reaction. In my experience, there is an overemphasis by veterinarians and pet store owners on allergy symptoms rather than on investigating *why* and *how* the body reacts as it does. Often, the animal's symptoms are cyclic, changing from diet to diet, or from one conditioner to another, with medications (including allergy shots) used to suppress the resulting symptoms. With each cycle or season, the allergy response becomes worse and more difficult to treat. Tests are performed to identify specific allergens and every attempt is made to avoid these sources. Short-term relief is generally successful, as long as the body remains responsive to medication. Eventually, more serious allergies and other progressive diseases can develop.

Sophisticated skin and blood tests may be able to ascertain what is happening with the body's biochemical processes, but unfortunately, they rarely identify a true allergen. Only detective work on the part of the owner will uncover the culprit.

Blood work identifies the presence of various markers, such as histamines, lymphocytes, and antibodies to specific allergens (i.e., beef proteins). These markers show us that the immune system has marshaled a defense. They do not show us if the specific source tested is the actual allergen, or whether a toxic level of waste *from that source* is the allergen. For example, if beef protein is compromised (i.e., contains diseased tissue or non-digestible sources of protein such as hide or hooves) and the body had a difficult time digesting and assimilating it, then a higher quantity of toxic waste products would circulate in the blood. These toxins could also trigger a release of histamines, but the blood work would only be able to reveal beef as the allergen. A standard course of treatment would recommend the elimination of beef and beef by-products. This same pet, now supported holistically and presented with a higher-quality beef diet, will no longer exhibit symptoms.

This dilemma is at the crux of the allergy firestorm. In holistic circles, this process is known as a "sensitivity." For example, if your body is constantly covered in filth, it will eventually begin to respond to the filth, possibly resulting in the skin tissue becoming sensitive and irritated. Imagine that the body is submersed in a vat of filth ten hours per day, and the prescribed treatment for the resultant skin problems was a fifteen-minute shower and the application of medicated creams two or three times per day. How quickly do you think the skin would heal completely? Would it ever have a chance to completely heal, being exposed daily, for hours at a time to the very source of irritation?

The same holds true for filth inside the body: It remains in contact with the mucous membranes in the respiratory or the digestive tract, irritating the nervous system, weakening the immune system, and imbalancing the glandular system. The eliminatory system becomes overburdened and unable to filter (detoxify) this filth.

As a holistic practitioner, I fully understand this vicious cycle and why it occurs in so many pets today. Our pets are constantly bombarded with chemicals, by-products, vaccinations, etc., and subjected to life in a symbolic "vat" of filth. When a substance is not easily broken down and absorbed and eliminated by the body, a build-up of waste results. An overabundance of waste results in toxic levels, which stimulates the body's immune system to release agents to corral and eliminate the culprit (hence, the positive results in blood work-ups). But the condition cannot be reversed through repeated suppression of symptoms with chemical treatment. This cycle of suppressing the symptoms sentences thousands of pets to a lifetime of pain and suffering and perpetuates the myth that allergies cannot be cured.

THE UNDERLYING IMBALANCE

The diagnosis of "allergies" has steadily increased over the past ten years. In 1986 a valuable book identified several important factors to aid in the understanding and treatment of allergy sensitivities. In *Pet Allergies: Remedies for an Epidemic*, Alfred J. Plechner, DVM, and Martin Zucker described how commercial pet food ingredients can undermine general health. The authors also emphasized the fallout of improper breeding practices, which result in genetically crippled animals and rampant disease. They discussed the safe use of steroids and hormones in specific cases. For the most part, the veterinarians and breeders for whom it was written ignored this book.

Pet food companies have manufactured new and improved diets for allergy symptoms based on new sources of animal protein instead of the traditional beef, meat meal and bone meal, pork by-products, and other animal by-products. Unfortunately, these new sources are not too different from the old: lamb, lamb meal and bone meal, poultry by-products, fish by-products and other animal by-products! The use of chemicals in pet foods is still rampant. If anything, there are even more chemicals and by-products being fed to our pets today under the guise of a "natural" or "anti-allergen" product! The fundamental quality of the diet is still sadly lacking.

Breeders continue to breed animals known to have a predisposition towards allergies. Veterinarians continue to use prednisone, antihistamines, and antibiotics, but misunderstand the true benefit of these medications in some of these allergy-related cases. Plechner and Zucker describe how the use of corticosteroids can reestablish cortisol levels (a deficiency of which is seen in many allergy-suffering pets), which stimulates and strengthens the immune system and promotes reversal of symptoms. They identified simple blood work which could be used to determine which animals could truly profit from steroids (to reverse a deficiency), and which animals would benefit from hormone therapy, instead of using the shotgun approach and giving these medications to any pet with similar symptoms. This method of identification is extremely helpful in those pets with true deficiencies that should be treated chemically. In the remaining animals, the immune system would have an opportunity to be stimulated naturally through nutritional, herbal, and homeopathic supplementation, rather than further burdened by medications not truly needed.

The quality and freshness of the ingredients in food play a role in triggering an allergic response. It is not necessarily the ingredient itself that is the allergen. Certainly, one should always seek to eliminate a food ingredient which may be an allergen, but a greater focus on the body's ability to properly digest and assimilate nutrition, eliminate waste, and repair and maintain healthy cells for a strong immune system is essential to the elimination of your pet's allergies.

Even if medication is needed, your pet's lifestyle can be enriched through holistic animal care. You will succeed if you honor life as nature's gift to your animal and use a holistic style to fully realize your animal's self-curative potential.

What Is Holistic Animal Care?

Rather than simply addressing an animal's symptoms, holistic animal care addresses the whole body, including body, mind, spirit, and even the environment. Different health modalities are used in a synergistic way to help stimulate, strengthen, and support the body's own biological processes and natural defenses.

Nutrition, which can often be the deciding factor between health and disease, is central to holistic care. Despite the number of drugs or natural remedies given to a pet, if the pet is not receiving adequate nutrition, it will be lacking the basic tools with which to support its own recovery.

Nutrition is also the cornerstone of a modality known as naturopathy. Defined by a medical dictionary as "a drugless system of therapy by the use of physical forces, such as air, light, water, heat, massage, etc.," naturopathy is a comprehensive approach which emphasizes supporting the body's physical attempts to eliminate disease. Naturopaths believe that a major cause of disease is an excessive build-up of toxic materials (often due to improper eating and lack of exercise) which clog the eliminatory system. Various techniques are used to clean out (detoxify) the body and stimulate the reversal of symptoms and disease. The cleansing process is supported with high-quality nutrition, proper food combining (to stimulate and aid digestion), and nutritional supplements and herbs.

Herbs have been used extensively by every culture since ancient times to stimulate healing. It is widely believed that people began using herbs after observing wild animals instinctively select appropriate herbs when they are ill. Herbalists use specific herbal leaves, roots, bark, flowers, and seeds to assist the healing process, primarily by helping to detoxify the body. Herbs provide a slower and deeper action than pharmaceutical drugs.

Another modality which also provides a slower and deeper action is homeopathy. Sometimes nutrition or herbs can begin the cleansing process and support the body so that it can cure itself. But often it is the homeopathic remedy that can stimulate the deeper levels of healing. The homeopathic system is safe, its basic principles are elegantly simple, and homeopathic remedies have been exhaustively researched and used successfully for hundreds of years.

The German physician, Samuel Hahnemann, founded homeopathy in the late 1700s. The basic principle of homeopathy is "Like will cure like." This principle was recognized by the ancient Chinese masters of the healing arts, Hindu sages, as well as Western history's most noted physicians and alchemists, Hippocrates and Paracelsus. Hahnemann's "provings"—that a substance that can mimic symptoms helps cure the symptoms as well—revolutionized the understanding of symptoms and disease. Trained as a physician, Hahnemann had treated symptoms as the unhealthy responses of the body that should be suppressed. He later learned that symptoms can be positive, adaptive responses to stressors that the body experiences. Hahnemann recognized that symptoms represented the body's effort to heal itself, and therefore our aim should be to stimulate instead of suppress the body's own defenses.

Hahnemann noted certain similarities between symptoms produced by some diseases and the very drugs used to treat them. From this he formed his "Law of Similars," postulating that a disease could be cured by whatever medicine produces similar symptoms when given to a healthy person. The beauty of homeopathic treatment is that it cooperates, rather than competes, with the body's own efforts to regain health.

A simplified example of how homeopathy works is that of bee venom. We know that a bee sting will cause swelling, fluid accumulation, redness of the skin, pain, and soreness that is accentuated by the application of heat or pressure. Sensitive animals will also experience mental (emotional) symptoms such as apathy, stupor, listlessness, or the opposite, whining and fearfulness. If a homeopathically prepared *dilute solution* of bee venom (known as Apis) is given to a pet with these symptoms—even if they are caused by something other than a bee sting—the condition will soon begin to clear up. The key is that the symptoms are quite similar to what the remedy, in its undiluted state, would create. Flower essences (which balance emotional states) and tissue cell salts (which support physiological processes) act similarly, by stimulating the body's own natural healing and homeostasis.

THE HOLISTIC PET

A healthy, holistically reared pet is in a state of balance which manifests on three interrelated levels: the physical, the emotional, and the environmental. A healthy pet experiences physical vitality and is free from physiological malfunction, displays emotional clarity resulting in good behavior and happiness, and receives (as well as contributes) joy, love, and security in their living environment.

This animal is the opposite of a chemically reared pet, who is often found to be in a state of imbalance or dis-ease. This animal lacks physical vitality and suffers from chronic symptoms due to physiological malfunction, displays emotional stress resulting in negative behavior, and often lives in a physically toxic environment. Since it is impossible to have one organ system affected without it in turn affecting the other organ systems, a system that is not in balance is more susceptible to assault from toxins or allergens.

Holistic animal care is simple and safe to use. *Treat the body well and the body will be well.* By providing the body with sufficient amounts of high-quality food, enhanced by the correct supplements, and holistic modalities when appropriate—the body will remain in a healthy balance. If the balanced body is assaulted by certain substances which create an imbalance, it has the strength to trigger the curative process and reestablish its balance.

THE ALLERGIC PET

Some pets who are born genetically compromised develop allergies to certain foods, such as mother's milk. Most of the pets who were not born genetically compromised also suffer from allergies because they are exposed to chemicals and an emotionally and/or physically toxic environment. Chemicals alter the body's primary biological functions, place undue stress on vital organs and glands necessary for proper immune function, and destroy healthy tissue. Allergic pets have often been exposed to:

- standard commercial pet foods
- artificial treats
- shotgun medications (the indiscriminate use of "standard" medications)
- excessive vaccinations and yearly boosters
- toxic cleaning and pest-control products (especially collars or monthly drug doses)
- environmental pollution (without the benefit of regular detoxification)
- an emotionally and/or physically stressful living environment (past and present)

Commercial Foods Increase Susceptibility to Allergies

Commercial pet diets and treats are the primary reason pets develop all types of allergies, including food allergies. But it should be noted that the quality of the ingredient can do more harm and is more likely to trigger a response than the ingredients themselves. The standard use of by-products and meat sources unfit for human consumption severely limits the pet's ability to digest and properly assimilate nutrients. The use of artificial colors or flavors, chemical preservatives, nitrates, and rancid animal fats also interferes with digestion. Poorly digested matter becomes harder to eliminate, causing a backup of old fecal material in the bowel, which further prevents assimilation of vital nutrients.

We can call this the screen door effect. Here in the desert where I live, we love screen doors and the ventilation that they provide. But we also struggle with blowing dirt and on the few days of the season when we get rain, my screen door can become caked with dirt. If I go out and brush it off right away there is not much of a problem, but if I wait a day or two the dirt can harden, especially if it rains again. Rain adheres the top layers of dirt more firmly onto the previous ones, creating an adobe mud effect, where the dirt becomes so hard that it cannot be brushed away and actually begins to block the flow of air.

This is similar to what is happening inside a poorly maintained colon. Imagine the colon as the screen door to the body and the nutrients are the air. As improperly digested matter moves into the colon, and because complete evacuation is not always encouraged (mostly pets lack exercise, and can't always go outside to have a bowel movement), old fecal material begins to "collect." This material lines the walls of the colon, and chemicals (such as ethoxyquin, a commonly used pet food preservative that prohibits moisture absorption) make the feces so dry they cannot move down the colon. This drying also affects the size and hardness of the stools.

Most companies try to convince you that these stools only mean their food is more "digestible with less waste to pick up." What do you think a medical doctor would say to you, if you described your own stools as coming out like that? Certainly, a better-quality food will produce less stool volume (generally due to less fillers *first*, and better digestibility *second*), but it should not be from lack of moisture in the stool.

As old fecal material builds up inside the colon, the "screen door effect" begins. It becomes harder and harder for the body to clean out this material on its own. This interferes with the body's ability to absorb (or "ventilate") nutrients from digested matter in the intestines into the bloodstream to use for distribution among the body's hungry cells and energy-depleted organ systems.

The harder the pet food ingredients are to break down and process, and the more chemicals that are present, the more stress is placed on the body to function. The harder the body has to work, the quicker it breaks down and falls apart. With improper digestion and assimilation, the body cannot utilize nutrients that are vital to proper biological processes such as immunity (resistance to allergens). Improper digestion and assimilation also leads to a build-up of general waste (toxins) in the body, which subsequently places a huge burden upon the eliminatory organs. As the liver and kidneys become burdened, the body attempts to detoxify through the largest eliminatory organ it has, the skin, which leads to the development of skin and coat problems normally associated with allergies. Additionally, the lymph system and endocrine system are overstimulated, possibly leading to the development of a deeper, more serious disease such as cancer.

Chemicals in Non-Foods

A pet may also be exposed to chemicals and irritants in other, non-dietary, forms. Whether the irritant is a chemical-based breath mint given as a treat, an annual vaccination booster, an artificially perfumed shampoo, a medicated skin treatment, flea or tick control products, household cleaning agents, long-term medication—any or all of the above can have a detrimental effect on your animal's health. If you think of the healthy body as a balanced scale, and you keep adding these chemicals to one side, the scale remains off-balance. But if you add good nutrition and minimize the build-up of chemicals on the other side, this scale stays in balance.

OTHER FACTORS CREATING IMBALANCE IN A PET

It is important to recognize and address other factors which may cause imbalance and interfere with homeostasis. Structural imbalances are often a prime cause of dis-ease. Old injuries or genetic malfunctions, such as rheumatoid arthritis, can place stress on certain organ systems. A build-up of calcium deposits and joint or spinal inflammation may also put pressure on the nerves that are involved with digestive organs such as the stomach. This pressure can interfere with the normal function of the stomach and lead to improper digestion and assimilation of nutrients. Often, addressing these structural problems will help to reverse the "allergy" condition. Chiropractic adjustments, massage, acupressure, and acupuncture can all be beneficial tools in your fight against your animal's allergies.

Another factor that can also cause imbalance is a stressful environment. Have you ever "felt butterflies in your stomach" and experienced a loose bowel due to a stressful situation? Pets who often experience extreme emotions (fear, nervousness, and tension) are also more likely to suffer from digestive problems and glandular imbalances, which may exacerbate allergy symptoms. Sources of environmental stress include family changes such as vacations, members leaving or dying, divorce or new births, new jobs, etc. The pituitary, adrenal, and thyroid glands all may be injured by chronic emotional stress. These glands are associated with the fight-or-flight reaction to negative stimulus which is common to all living things. A safe and nurturing environment will ensure your pet's emotional well-being. The use of nutritional supplementation and remedies, especially flower essences, to re-balance the emotions, can often be the key to a more complete physical healing.

When an animal is out of balance, waste builds up not only in the colon but also in the bloodstream and other eliminatory organs. Urea, a waste product of meat protein metabolism, can cause allergy-related conditions, and accounts for the high number of pets who test positive for meat allergies. The poorer the quality of meat, and the more difficult it is to digest, the more waste is produced during digestion. Urea toxicity manifests itself through certain notable symptoms:

- known or suspected allergies to beef, pork, meat, meat by-products, or meat meal
- excessive licking and chewing of paws, resulting in lick granuloma
- prickly heat-type rashes, itchy skin, with or without small pimples or pustules
- excessive loss of hair, or coat condition

- foul-smelling breath, flatulence, and/or stool
- increased fatty tumor, cyst, or cancerous tumor production
- liver, pancreatic, gallbladder, and kidney dysfunction
- weakened immune responses, especially chronic skin infections
- premature aging with or without chronic muscular pain and/or arthritic symptoms
- parasitic infestation, especially fleas and ticks (which feed off of skin-eliminated waste)
- neurological issues, including seizures
- aggression and other behavioral problems

Yeast is another nasty ingredient found in the majority of commercial pet diets, treats, supplements, flea and tick control products, and even many pet medications. Yeast, which is noted for its anti-flea and tick properties, is in practically everything! A cheap filler ingredient, it does provide some B vitamins, minerals, amino acids, and natural flavor to products, but it is mostly used to increase the food's volume.

The most common form of yeast is brewer's yeast, which is actually a waste product which has most of its nutrients eliminated during the brewing process. Yeast was long touted as a good source of nutrients, but we are now finding that this is not so. Nutritional yeast, a cultivated product, is nutritionally superior to and tastier than brewer's yeast, but it still is not the best source of nutrients and, like brewer's yeast, it can be difficult to digest. Adequate levels of B vitamins are only available through supplements. It would take far too much yeast to provide an equivalent amount. Moreover, excessive yeast clogs the liver and increases general toxicity. According to recent veterinary research, animals are more likely to be allergic to yeast than to most other food sources.

Humans also do not digest yeast well. This poor digestion places an additional burden on the liver, resulting in skin conditions. Chinese medicine recognizes the correlation between the liver and the skin. Yeast supplementation, prescribed by vets and alternative practitioners, may initially improve pets' skin, but then the pets' symptoms often become more intense and more difficult to treat, which results in liver toxicity symptoms as well. I always recommend detoxification and the total elimination of yeast and sugar (which compounds yeast toxicity) from animals' diets for six weeks. Other than a daily multiple vitamin/mineral supplement (high in B vitamins) nothing else was used to treat their skin condition, yet it would quickly resolve on its own.

One of my human clients, who had suffered from oozing skin eruptions for years and had been diagnosed as having chronic liver problems, tested positive for a yeast allergy. Three months later, under my guidance, she was given a clean bill of health and had a negative reaction for a yeast allergy! We then reintroduced yeast into her diet and she never had another flare-up, as long as she did not deviate from her holistic lifestyle.

Yeast toxicity manifests itself in certain symptoms, which include:

- known or suspected allergies to yeast or yeast-containing foods such as dry kibble
- ear infections, eye discharges, and upper respiratory problems, including asthma
- excessive licking and chewing of the body and face-rubbing
- hot spots, itchy skin, with or without small pimples or pustules
- slower healing of skin problems
- excessive loss of feathers, fur, or coat condition
- foul-smelling breath, flatulence, and/or stool (especially off-colored stools with mucus)

- increased fatty tumor, cyst, or cancerous tumor production
- poor digestion and assimilation of other nutrients
- blood sugar instability
- high levels of liver enzymes and eosinophils (represents a damaged liver)
- liver, spleen, gallbladder, and/or pancreatic dysfunction including diabetes
- weakened immune responses, especially chronic skin infections
- premature aging, with or without digestive symptoms
- increased sensitivies to pollution, vaccinations, and chemicals in general
- aggression, fearful-aggressive, or fearful behavior in certain pets
- parasitic infestation, especially fleas and ticks (which feed off of skin-eliminated waste)

Research on flea and tick infestations has determined that garlic is more powerful as an antiparasitic agent by itself than when it is used in combination with yeast, or when yeast alone is used. A clean diet greatly reduces the waste eliminated through the skin. This waste is the very thing that attracts a flea or tick to the body in the first place and then feeds them. Old fecal material in the colon also attracts and feeds internal parasites such as worms.

As urea, metabolized yeast, and other excessive waste builds up in the body, undue stress is placed upon vital organs. First, the ability to break down ingredients is reduced, waste begins to circulate, and fewer nutrients are available to stimulate the body's own defenses. Next, the eliminatory, lymphatic, and immune systems become burdened. Chronic symptoms develop—notably those diagnosed as "allergies"—and suppression of the symptoms is initiated. Once medication is stopped the symptoms return and the cycle continues. Ultimately, there is organ and gland malfunction, possibly leading to an early death.

Any pet suffering from allergies, sensitivities, or toxicity (all of which may be labeled allergies) can benefit from holistic animal care. Regardless of the symptoms, the underlying causes are fundamentally the same. A wholesome, toxic-free approach to diet and environment can not only prevent an allergy-type symptom, but can also reverse it more quickly and effectively than the further application of chemicals.

How to Reverse Your Pet's Allergies Holistically

In order to address allergies successfully by completely reversing their symptoms, a holistic animal care lifestyle must be followed, or you run the risk of suppressing symptoms only temporarily. Fasting and detoxification is an important first step. These processes help prepare the body for further rebalancing, and ultimately for healing. Changing to a natural, high-quality diet, supplemented with nutritional, herbal, and homeopathic products, provides the necessary foundation to help facilitate specific curative responses.

Treating allergies without first addressing a possible underlying nutritional imbalance is a waste of time. Diet may be a causative factor. Many treats, and even so-called "natural" supplements, are full of fillers such as yeast, chemicals, artificial flavors and colors. Look carefully at what you are feeding your pet. Re-balance a home-cooked diet, or find a better-quality commercial diet, and your pet's allergies may be reversed.

To introduce a dietary change and to kick off a successful allergy-relief program, begin by imposing a short twenty-four-hour period of fasting. Many people associate fasting with deliberately starving their pet, yet this couldn't be further from the truth. Fasting can save your pet's life!

Fasting encourages the body to detoxify and re-balance. Old fecal material is expelled from the colon. Vital eliminatory organs—the kidneys and liver—are given a respite from processing waste, thus allowing a deeper processing of backed-up toxins to take place. Digestion and elimination, necessary processes for the uptake of nutrients and therapeutic substances such as herbs, are improved. The immune system, which helps the body resist allergens, is strengthened. And, finally, the overall condition of your pet is improved.

The fasting methods we will explore are very safe and gentle. People are bothered most when their pets look at them pleadingly at dinnertime. It is true that twenty-five percent of that pleading look may be caused by hunger, but you should know that the other seventy-five percent is definitely an attempt to control you. Pets, particularly dogs, are experts at controlling their masters. To avoid the pleading look during fasting, do something that's fun with your pet during their usual dinnertime. Bring home a new kitty toy (but, please, not out of guilt!), or take your canine friend out for a fifteen-minute walk. These activities will not only occupy your and your pet's minds, but will also provide you both with much-needed exercise. If your pet cannot be fasted because of its physical condition, homeopathic detoxification works well by itself.

In order to encourage elimination still further, you can add a homeopathic remedy during the twenty-four-hour period of fasting. This combination of fasting along with a homeopathic remedy is the fastest way to detoxify a pet's body. If you use the homeopathic remedy alone or the fasting alone, the process will take longer.

Anyone who has tried to clean with a dirty sponge can relate to the fact that once that sponge has been rinsed out, it becomes more effective at doing its job. Even a short twenty-four-hour fast with homeopathic support can make a world of difference. Detoxification makes for better digestion and better assimilation of the vital nutrients necessary to help stimulate healing and strengthening. Without proper detoxification, you are severely limiting the body's overall curative potential.

Once the detoxification process has occurred, usually within the first six to eight weeks, you will see a reversal of symptoms. In over seventy-five percent of cases I have observed, this detoxification of the body, plus dietary changes and basic nutritional support, effectively ended the pet's "allergy" suffering days.

In the remaining twenty-five percent of cases, including those with true allergies or chronic debilitating dis-ease, the judicious use of homeopathic, herbal, and nutritional supplementation in a *continuing* course of treatment will definitely affect the strengthening of the animal's constitution and improve, or eventually eliminate, their condition. With these cases, it can often take several seasons to build up the body sufficiently to eliminate the allergies completely.

This is why a holistic lifestyle should be followed rather than relying on the suppression of symptoms. Addressing your pet's allergic reactions holistically is the quickest, most effective way to reverse an allergy (or any underlying) condition. With a systematic detoxification and strengthening program, the underlying condition continues to improve, although the improvement will not be so obvious. Don't stop detoxification and supplementation as soon as symptoms have been suppressed. If you do, the body will become burdened again (because it has a predisposition to this weakness), and will again respond to allergens or stress.

For pets with true allergies or chronic dis-ease, the results of an ongoing holistic animal care program can be miraculous. As each season passes, the body will become stronger and less sensitive to allergens and toxins. The animal will exhibit less severe symptoms that become easier to treat, and there will be faster resolution. In those animals that have been genetically or environmentally predisposed to deeper dis-ease, holistic animal care will minimize degenerative possibilities and maximize what curative potential there is.

Before starting a fasting program, check with your veterinarian. Perhaps your pet has diabetes and must maintain their blood sugar with food as well as insulin. Perhaps your veterinarian feels that your pet is too weak to fast. Maybe your pet has had a recent bout of minor infections. It is always wise to rely on a trusted medical opinion, especially if you have a veterinarian who supports your holistic lifestyle.

There are two methods to fasting that I recommend. The biggest difference between the two is the condition of your pet prior to starting the fast.

THE STANDARD FAST

The standard method of fasting is used for pets with acute or chronic allergic responses who are otherwise in good health. These animals can adhere to a straight fast. Age makes no difference, as I have seen fasting succeed with a struggling one-week-old kitten or a fourteen-year-old dog.

Day One

Feed your pet breakfast as you normally would on the morning you are to begin the fast. Simply eliminate the evening meal altogether. Be sure to provide plenty of fresh drinking water. Provide fun-filled activity in fresh air and sunshine, twice during the first day, followed by a damp terry cloth rubdown. Be sure not to overtire or place undue stress on your pet.

Day Two—Breaking the Fast

The following morning (after twenty-four hours of fasting) feed your pet one-half its usual breakfast. To make this process really special, break the fast with cooked oatmeal—

it will absorb impurities in the digestive tract. To the oatmeal, you can add a teaspoon or two of raw honey, encapsulated garlic oil (raw garlic can be too harsh at this point), and some type of fresh green extract such as barley grass or spirulina, which can be very soothing and cleansing to the digestive system after fasting. Cats prefer tuna water for flavor. Supplements can also be added back into the diet at this time.

Provide exercise in the fresh air and sunshine twice on this second day, followed by a damp terry cloth rubdown. Remember to provide plenty of water, and be sure not to overtire or stress out your pet. For dinner, feed the normal quantity (and, hopefully, better quality) of food.

This is also a good fasting protocol to follow on a weekly basis to help maintain general health and well-being. You will quickly find what suits you and your own animal's needs regarding this weekly fast. Remember that exercise is very important at all times, but especially so during cleansing to help move toxins out of the body by further stimulating the eliminatory organs. The terry cloth rubdown also helps to stimulate the skin (the largest eliminatory organ) as it continues to process waste from the body's detoxification. If an odor is present during fasting, mix one-quarter cup of baking soda to one gallon of warm, purified water and rinse off the pet's body with this solution, and then dry it with a towel. The baking soda will help to neutralize the odor and balance the skin's pH, reducing any itching. Avoid using tap water, as it contains chlorine (a known skin irritant that will increase itching), which will be absorbed back into the skin. If tap water is the only available water, boil it for fifteen minutes to help evaporate the chlorine. Be sure to let it cool down before using. A cut-up lemon boiled in the water for twenty minutes, then strained, makes a wonderful additional deodorizer and acts as a disinfectant as well.

Generally, a standard twenty-four-hour fast is sufficient, but you may choose to follow it for two to three days longer if your pet was suddenly overcome by allergies, is fighting an infection, has been on a very poor-quality diet, or has not been eating well.

EXTENDED STANDARD FAST
Day One
Use the same protocol as the standard fast.

Day Two (and possibly Day Three, Day Four)
Provide fun-filled activity in fresh air and sunshine twice during this day of fasting, followed by a damp terry cloth rubdown. Be especially sure not to overtire or place undo stress on your pet. Apple juice or vegetable juices (carrot, celery, or parsnip is best—avoid tomato juice) may be given in small amounts during the day, approximately one-quarter cup per twenty-five pounds of body weight per day. Do not overdo! These juices can also be frozen into small ice cubes for your pet's enjoyment during warmer months.

Breaking Fast Day
Break this fast with one-quarter of your pet's normal quantity of food in the morning, and the same (one-quarter) quantity for dinner. Both meals should be the cooked oatmeal. A little fruit or vegetable fiber (from juicing) can be also added to the oatmeal and future meals.

Second Day of Breaking Fast
Feed one-half of normal rations in the morning and evening of the second day. Mix your pet's new natural diet fifty-fifty with cooked oatmeal.

Third Day of Breaking Fast

Feed full rations of a natural diet of your choice at breakfast and dinner. This is a good time to introduce fresh fruits and vegetables to your pet's diet on a regular basis.

THE ALTERNATIVE FASTING METHOD

This method may be more appropriate for pets with allergies who also struggle with other serious conditions, such as cancer or diabetes, or who are very debilitated to begin with and require additional nutritional and/or herbal support. This method is used primarily to avoid huge dips in blood sugar and additional stress on the animal's biochemical balance. For these pets, fasting should be limited to twenty-four hours. Actually, it is easier and almost as beneficial for the body to complete several twenty-four hour fasts within a few weeks, even if there are only a few days break in-between each twenty-four hour fast, rather than three or four consecutive days of fasting. This alternative fasting period can be a bit more complicated, but well worth it to your pet.

Day One

Feed your pet its usual breakfast. For the evening meal substitute a vegetable broth. To make this broth, grate equal amounts of fresh, raw carrots, beets, parsley, parsnips, spinach, and kale to make up a total of one cup of combined vegetables. Add grated vegetables to four cups of boiling water (avoid tap water) and simmer on low until all the vegetables are very soft, about twenty to thirty minutes. Separate the cooked vegetables and refrigerate to be used later. Refrigerate the broth in a well-sealed container.

Feed your pet one-half cup of broth per twenty pounds of body weight, per meal. You may give one or two additional meals of this broth during the fasting, if your animal seems to be very hungry, but do not overfeed in one sitting. Prior to feeding, warm the broth—but never in the microwave, which will destroy any available nutrients. Cold broth may upset sensitive stomachs and lacks palatability. Prior to feeding the broth, give your pet any oral supplements or medications prescribed to be given with food.

Break Alternative Fast Day

The next morning, feed your pet one-half the amount of broth you used during the preceding day, adding one-quarter the normal ration of food. Cooked oatmeal may be a good alternative to regular food during this fast-breaking period, especially if there is a lot of colon cleansing needed. Repeat the morning menu for the evening meal.

Second Day of Breaking the Alternative Fast

Feed one-half the amount of broth you used during the fast and add one-quarter the normal ration of food *or* one-eighth ration of food and one-eighth ration of cooked oatmeal. For the evening meal feed three-quarters the normal ration of food (no broth).

Third Day of Breaking the Alternate Fast

Introduce the full ration of your pet's natural diet at each meal.

This protocol will allow the body to begin detoxification without too much stress. When in doubt as to which process should be followed, it might be best to use the alternative fasting protocol. In a pinch, try cutting back twenty-five percent to fifty percent of their standard meal with the addition of nutritional supplements, herbal extracts, vegetable and fruit juices—which will also serve to stimulate a deeper elimination, without upsetting their metabolism.

SUPPORTIVE PHYTOCHEMICALS

The top detoxifying herbs, vegetables, and fruits (gentle enough to use during the fasting period) are:

Milk Thistle is good for liver cleansing and support.

Dandelion is an effective blood purifier and general organ cleanser.

Burdock Root helps remove catabolic waste from cellular activity.

Slippery Elm is very soothing to inflamed colon tissues and helps settle the stomach.

Yucca is a natural anti-inflammatory, supports circulation, and reduces discomfort.

Garlic is anti-bacterial, anti-viral, anti-fungal, and anti-parasitic.

Kombu is a sea vegetable which alkalizes the body and purifies the blood of fats.

Spirulina is high in chlorophyll and aids enzyme production and digestion.

Carrots are trace mineral-rich, high in vitamins, and alkalize the body.

Beets provide several supportive nutrients, texture, and flavor.

Parsnips provide wonderful support for detoxifying the kidneys.

Spinach is an excellent source of nutrients and trace minerals.

Celery is trace mineral-rich, high in vitamins, alkalizing, and flavorful to pets.

Parsley is trace mineral-rich, oxygenating to the blood, and helps detoxify odors.

Ginger	can help the digestive system, reduce gas, and aids hypertension.
Apples	provide needed energy while supporting detoxification.
Cranberries	are very high in Vitamin C, and help flush urinary tract waste.
Papaya	rebalances and aids digestion, and helps flush wastes.

Avoid highly acidic vegetables like tomatoes and onions (which can be deadly to pets), or difficult-to-digest ingredients like cabbage. Also avoid the use of harsh fibers such as psyllium, which can further irritate and damage sensitive intestinal tissues. Although a good ingredient for producing bulk and encouraging elimination, psyllium's negative side effects outweigh its benefits during detoxification.

HOMEOPATHIC DETOXIFICATION

Homeopathic detoxification encourages elimination and works well when combined with fasting or used alone. One or several individual homeopathic remedies may be chosen, based on your pet's individual needs, or you may find that one of the many available combination remedies will work just as well. For detoxification it is best to work within the lower potencies, X's to low C's. Homeopathic detoxification should be used daily for no less than two weeks, preferably six to eight weeks. Give one daily dose at bedtime for most cases, or one dose upon rising and again at bedtime for more chronic cases.

Sometimes it is advisable to allow an initial build-up of the remedy by frequent dosing. Give one dose every fifteen minutes for the first hour (four times) when beginning detoxification and at any other time you feel that your pet might need a little extra detoxifying boost. You cannot over-dose your pet. Each repeated dose enhances the effect. (See "Symptom Reversal," for more details on homeopathic dosing.)

After the initial detoxification process, a maintenance program can be initiated on a weekly basis: a single weekly dose at bedtime to help process current waste build-up, stimulate proper kidney and liver function, and support general good health. It does not mean that homeopathic detoxification should be used in lieu of proper feeding, supplementing, and care. It should be used only as a support to biological functions such as digestion and elimination.

Homeopathic Remedies for Detoxification

Antimonium Crudum is good for gout-like symptoms with gastric weaknesses.

Arsenicum Album is used for general detoxification, and rebalances the liver and spleen.

Berberis Vulgaris is good for a gouty constitution, particularly for a pet with a history of poor nutrition.

Bryonia helps digestive problems that contribute to waste build-up.

Cadium Sulph balances basic dis-ease that has gastric involvement.

Carduus Marianus supports the vascular system, gallbladder, and liver.

Chelidonium Majus is a liver remedy for degenerative diseases.

Hydrastis improves liver action and stimulates the immune system.

Juniperus Communis	encourages kidney elimination.
Solidago Vira	supports kidney detoxification.
Taraxacum	is used for bilious attacks and flatulence associated with cleansing.
Nux Vomica	helps to counter nausea, irritability, digestive disturbances, and liver congestion sometimes associated with the detoxification process.

Nux Vomica is often the first remedy that homeopaths choose to establish equilibrium of biological functions and to counteract many chronic effects. It should always be included, regardless of what other remedies are chosen. The best homeopathic combinations for detoxification on the market today include this remedy. I have used *Arsenicum Album* and *Nux Vomica* to reverse many acute toxic reactions (including pesticide poisonings). When in doubt, this is a sound combination to try.

WHAT TO EXPECT DURING DETOXIFICATION

Since detoxification is the process of ridding the body of waste, waste will present itself during the detoxification process. Sometimes the very symptoms you are trying to address with the cleansing process are aggravated. This is a good sign! Called a *curative response*, it is a clear indicator that the body has been stimulated into cleansing. Curative responses are a natural part of detoxification and are vital to strengthening and rebalancing the body. When this response occurs, the first impulse many people have is to run to the veterinarian to get a drug to suppress the resulting symptoms. Don't do it!

In striving to reach your pet's fullest curative potential, it is vital to the process that symptoms be *supported* rather than *suppressed*. More so than at any other time, suppression of these symptoms—even through the use of holistic animal care, rather than drugs—will only strive to force the underlying imbalance even deeper. The use of chemicals and medications—especially steroids and antibiotics at this point—will also severely burden the body and limit the cleansing process.

Sometimes people will prematurely terminate the cleansing process because they fear the return or worsening of their pet's symptoms. Although symptoms may have been suppressed through veterinary or natural methods, if the cleansing process is terminated prematurely, you and your pet will eventually have to go through the process again if you can ever hope for true healing. It is best to address the symptoms gently (naturally), while continuing detoxification. Many things can be done to help minimize the aggravation (curative response) your pet experiences, without suppressing the cleansing and strengthening process. The safest, most effective way to support symptom aggravations is through the gentle modalities of nutritional supplements, homeopathy, flower essences, and herbs. (See "Symptoms: A to Z," to address specific symptoms.)

Please note that aggravations do not have to occur for the body to be detoxified. It is more common for the process to happen relatively easily, regardless of the pet's previous condition.

Pets who seemed to be healthy prior to detoxification can exhibit the worst symptoms, perhaps from an imbalance that was suppressed long ago. The bottom line is that you must be aware of your own pet's individual process and support that—regardless of any preconceived notions you may have had regarding what the process should be like. Each time the body experiences a curative response, which has been supported rather than suppressed, the body is strengthened, and the symptoms will return less frequently and less aggressively until eventually the symptoms are eliminated (reversed) completely.

Please, do not forget the power of love. Spend time nurturing your pet, even if only to respect their need to be quiet and sleep more during this process of symptom reversal. Such tenderness will certainly help minimize any stress they may be experiencing.

HINTS TO AID THE GENERAL DETOXIFICATION PROCESS

Provide plenty of pure water. Water is needed to help flush wastes as they are being eliminated. Avoid using tap water, which contains chlorine and chemicals (which may be too harsh for the kidneys to handle), or distilled water, which may facilitate too rapid a detoxification. Be sure that your pet's drinking water is always free of metals and sediments.

Groom daily. Grooming is necessary to brush away toxins that are being eliminated though the skin. This also stimulates circulation, further aiding elimination. Removal of old, dead skin also stimulates the growth of new, healthier coats. Wipe away any ear, eye, penile, vaginal, or anal discharges to avoid infections.

Provide daily exercise in fresh air and sunshine. This is necessary to encourage respiration, which supports the removal of deeper toxins. This also improves your pet's attitude, which supports healing. For indoor-only kitties, please provide a screened-in area where fresh air and sunshine can still be enjoyed.

Respect your pet's quiet times. Do so even if the pet's withdrawal from interaction with the family troubles you. It is normal for pets going through detoxification to sleep more, to continue the fasting process on their own when they need to, to become irritable, or to seek out warmer or cooler areas.

Avoid the use of all chemicals and drugs that are not absolutely necessary for sustaining life. They will severely interfere in the detoxification process and may even be more harmful to your pet during this time. As the cleansing process moves deeper into the body, your pet's reaction to these substances may be stronger than usual, and it is possible there may be an allergic reaction!

Avoid giving a vaccine booster within six weeks prior to, or after, a deep detoxification. The body may have a harder time detoxifying shortly after a vaccination, or may react even more strongly than usual.

Address symptom aggravations gently through the use of nutritional supplementation, homeopathy, flower essences, or herbs. This will allow the cleansing process to continue while keeping the symptoms from becoming too uncomfortable for your pet.

Keep track of your pet's progress to help you better understand the process they are going through. If you jot down a few notes each day, you will be less likely to scare yourself into thinking that it has been days since your pet last ate, when that simply isn't true.

On the one hand, if a discharge started three days ago and was clear but now has turned yellow, you will need to add natural antibiotics such as garlic or echinacea to fight off any possible infections that may have begun. Then you will want to keep track of how many days the discharge stays yellow, or how quickly it responded to the garlic, etc., so that you may seek out other support if needed. On the other hand, you might have noted that the discharge took two weeks to clear up—then returned in three weeks, but only took four days to clear up that second time. If it did not return for two months the next time—then you begin to see a pattern that indicates you are on the right track!

COMMON SYMPTOMS OF DETOXIFICATION

Abscesses can erupt during the detoxification process, especially around the chest and back. (See "Symptoms: A to Z.")

Dehydration can occur when there is excessive vomiting or diarrhea, causing an imbalance of nutrients and electrolytes. This will quickly shut down bodily functions, especially detoxification. To check for dehydration in a ferret, cat, or small dog, grab the skin from the back of the neck between your forefinger and thumb, pulling it gently upwards and then release it. In medium- to large-sized dogs, you can also press the side of the lip up and release it. The skin in either case should snap back into place within a second or two. If it takes longer, then dehydration is a problem. If the skin doesn't snap back at all (this is serious), consult your veterinarian immediately for subcutaneous fluid replacement therapy. In all other instances you can easily rehydrate your pet by encouraging them to drink water or by using a syringe, without a needle.

The average pet requires one ounce of water per pound of body weight per day—to remain fully hydrated. Additional water may be added to the food and drinking water can be flavored with sweetened fruit juice or tuna water to encourage drinking. Although commonly practiced, I do not recommend adding salt to the diet to increase thirst, as the negative side effects due to salt's naturally dehydrating properties are too counterproductive. Electrolyte solutions can be added to the water if the pet seems weakened by dehydration.

Diarrhea or constipation can sometimes occur, especially as old fecal materials are being processed, or as a side effect of general detoxification. One or two daily doses of homeopathic *Arsenicum* and *Nux Vomica*, helpful when nausea is also present, will generally firm up the stool while continuing to support elimination. If the diarrhea is severe or very watery, use this remedy more frequently: every fifteen minutes for the first hour and then every hour afterward, until the diarrhea is reversed. *Slippery Elm* is a soothing herb for the colon during and after a bout with diarrhea. In this case, use powdered *Slippery Elm* instead of the extract or tincture. To be certain that your animal is not dehydrating due to the loss of fluids through the diarrhea, watch how much water your pet drinks and check for the physical signs of dehydration.

Discharges from all orifices are normal during detoxification. These orifices are the routes that toxins can take directly out of the body. If your pet has a history of ear or eye irritations, nasal discharges, impacted anal glands (blocked discharge), mucous-coated stools, etc., you can expect an aggravation of these symptoms. Keep these areas clean, and utilize homeopathic remedies. *Arsenicum* is helpful as a general remedy, or you may want to explore others more directly suited to your pet's symptom. Regardless of where these discharges originate, *Calcarea Carbonica* is an excellent constitutional remedy for watery to thicker discharges, and *Pulsatilla* is suited for discharges that are thick and yellow to greenish in color.

Dry, flaky skin can be easily cared for with a good brushing, terry cloth rub, and the application of some *jojoba* or *tea tree oil conditioner.* Flaking of old discarded skin cells is a normal part of detoxification, as old tissue is being replaced by healthier skin. One or two doses of homeopathic *Sulphur* can also be very beneficial at this time. *M.S.M.* is a nutritional sulfur supplement that helps tissue repair and growth. The herb *Horsetail* also contains a high concentration of naturally occurring sulfur.

Frequent bathing can rob the skin of necessary oils, resulting in an excessive release of these oils, which are the body's attempt to rebalance the skin. Avoid bathing your pet more often than every few weeks.

Fever can be a good sign during detoxification, so long as the overall condition of the animal is stable. If you observe that your pet is severely exhausted, you may need to call a veterinarian. Fever supports detoxification, indicating that the body's defenses are working to burn up toxins and old viral or bacterial infections. If you suspect a fever after twenty-four hours of fasting or a few weeks of ongoing detoxification and dietary improvements, realize that it is a normal part of the detoxification process. However, support is needed to keep the fever from weakening the body while it does its job. Homeopathic remedies work best in this case. I highly recommend *Phosphorus*. If this fever is the result of an infection, increase garlic supplements, and add herbal products such as *Standardized Grapefruit Extract*, *Echinacea*, or *Golden Seal Root*, all excellent, safe, natural antibiotics. If the fever is high, especially with debilitating side effects, or lasts more than two days, seek out veterinary advice.

Flatulence can be a problem during cleansing, because old fecal material is being eliminated. Detoxification increases peristalsis (the muscular contractions inside the colon which move fecal matter along and help to further break it down). It's like turning over a well-decomposed compost heap so that the decayed material can be exposed and the odors released into the air. A good dose of *Arsenicum* and *Nux Vomica* will also help relieve flatulence.

Infections respond well to herbal support. Increase garlic supplements and add *Standardized Grapefruit Extract* (I highly recommend Nutri-Biotic's Citracidal), *Echinacea*, and/or *Golden Seal Root*. These are all excellent, safe, and highly effective natural antibiotics, which will work on the source of the infection and stimulate the immune system as well.

A homeopathic remedy that promotes drainage, or a combination of remedies for infections, can also be supportive in stimulating the body's defenses against the infection. Remedies that work well include *Antimonium Crudum* for skin infections with oozing and thick, yellow crusts, *Kal. Mur.* and *Kal. Phos.* (two types of tissue cell salts that aid in infections), or *Bioplasma* (the combination of all twelve tissue cell salts), and *Arsenicum*.

Loss of appetite. First determine if there is any fever present. Feed up to 100 mg. of *B-Complex vitamins* per day for cats or dogs. Many multiple vitamin/mineral products already include B vitamins, so check to see what you are already giving the animal first. A few doses of homeopathic *Arsenicum* (in general), *Nux Vomica* (if accompanied by one or more symptoms including nausea, vomiting, stool problems, flatulence), or *Belladonna* (if accompanied by nausea, empty retching and vomiting, as well as an aversion to drinking) works well. A dose or two daily of any of the above remedies, especially fifteen minutes prior to feeding, can also help stimulate appetite. Several flower essences, especially a combination formulation for minimizing stress, can often settle an animal enough so that it begins to regain some appetite. Always address emotional stress when appetite loss is evident, as it can often be a contributing factor.

Skin eruptions are the most common of detoxification symptoms. *Horsetail* and *Milk Thistle* are excellent herbs to use at this time, but homeopathic remedies such as *Apis* or *Sepia* (dry, rashy skin), *Rhus Tox.* (for clusters of tiny pimples that are extremely itchy), or *Graphites* (for scabby, oozy eruptions) work quickly to relieve irritation and discomfort. When in doubt try a dose of *Arsenicum* or *Sulphur*, both general skin remedies. *Antimonium Crudum* is best when staphylococcal or streptococcal infections are also present in the skin, but follow the above recommendations for infections as well.

Vomiting can also lead to dehydration and is often strictly symptomatic of detoxification rather than being an attempt to rid the stomach of an irritant. Therefore, since persistent vomiting will quickly exhaust your pet, it is appropriate to suppress this symptom quickly. Homeopathy works well, and is easier to administer, because it won't trigger vomiting as an herb would. For vomiting after eating, a combination of *Arsenicum* and *Nux Vomica* is effective. When vomiting occurs after drinking, use *Phosphorus* (with or without *Arsenicum*). Give one dose of each, every fifteen minutes for the first hour, then one dose every hour, until there has been no more vomiting for one hour. (See "Symptoms: A to Z.")

PROPER NUTRITION

The primary line of defense to prevent or reverse allergies is a sound nutritional program. After you have detoxified your pet's body, it is a perfect time to introduce a healthier diet.

Your pet's natural diet should consist of fresh, high-quality, easy to digest and assimilate ingredients. Since home cooking is optimal but not very practical for many people, you must be very careful to seek out a quality commercial product. Become an educated label reader, look beyond catchy terms such as "natural," "organic," "healthy," "allergy diet," and "human-grade quality," and ask the manufacturer directly to prove the quality of their products and guarantee their formula.

Seek out only Grade A or B meats (human grade) and avoid the four-D meats—dead, dying, diseased, or disabled animals not fit for human consumption. Four-D meats are those most commonly used in pet foods.

Grain by-products are also a big problem in commercial pet products. These include wheat millings, brewer's rice (leftovers from brewing), and flours. These inexpensive fillers are not only devoid of nutritional value, but also can severely compromise your pet's health. Manufacturers often include rancid and moldy grains in their products because they are cheaper. These poor-quality grain by-products add the possibility of a toxic reaction. Only Grade 1 or 2 grains (human grades) should be used, preferably whole ground, to ensure that their nutritional goodness remains intact.

People are often concerned that changing their pet's diet will only result in digestive upsets. This is true only if you are changing from a poor-quality or chemical-based diet to another one of the same sort. When you switch to a healthier, more natural diet, there should be no irritating ingredients to upset the balance. The only problems your pet might experience are soft stools and gas. This may happen because you may be overfeeding your pet with the new diet.

One cup of a grocery-store food is almost fifty percent filler! A better brand of grocery-type foods, even pet-shop pet food, or prescription diets can be just as bad. These may have less filler, but they will probably contain other types of by-products which may alter the volume of nutrients available in one cup. When switching to a higher-quality food, there generally is less filler, and therefore, feeding the same quantities (cup for cup) would result in overfeeding of the better brand. Carefully read and follow the manufacturer's recommendations for the food, and watch your pet carefully for the first few weeks to see how they react.

Overfeeding can often occur when people begin to cook for their pets. It is difficult to recommend one recipe that will suit everybody's needs, so I suggest that you seek out a well-researched book on natural pet care that include recipes.

Beware of feeding your pet raw meats. This can upset, rather than support your pet's condition. I believe this is because animals evolve to adapt to their environment. Our pets have been domesticated for so long that they have been altered to become processed food eaters and have lost the wild animal's ability to digest raw meat tissue, bone, hide, feathers, etc., on a regular basis. Even if you give your pet a digestive enzyme, it will probably still have to struggle to digest raw animal tissue.

If you prefer home-cooked foods to commercially processed pet foods, and you lightly cook the food so that all the enzymes and nutrients are not destroyed, cooking will break down the meat sufficiently, making it easier for your pet's digestive tract to handle.

Even with the best quality and balanced diet (commercial or home-cooked), nutritional supplementation is necessary to provide many nutrients now missing from our food chain. For instance, research indicates that fifty years ago spinach had up to eighty percent more nutritional value than today. This is true in varying degrees for other vegetables, grains, and fruits, as well as meats from animals fed "off the land." Our earth has been stripped of many of the naturally occurring micronutrients found in soil, which are then assimilated by plants. Years of overfarming, using toxic chemicals or fertilizers, and environmental pollution (such as acid rain), have taken their toll.

Even organic farming methods cannot guarantee that the produce is more nutritious, as it will take organic farmers approximately seventy-five years to completely return these nutrients back into the ground. Therefore, it is important that we supplement our animal's diets to ensure that they receive the fundamental nutrients required. Even pet foods which are "nutritionally complete" according to AAFCO (American Association of Feed Control Officers) guidelines still may not provide all that is needed for basic good health. For instance, the AAFCO standards require a certain amount of protein per cup of food, but that protein does not have to be digestible. So what good is it? This is also true for certain sources of Vitamin A or calcium, among other nutrients.

Proper nutrition not only includes quality, easy to digest foods, but also appropriate supplementation to support health. Such a regimen will stimulate your pet's curative potential, and also increase the ability to reverse any adverse symptom.

KEY INGREDIENTS FOR A HEALTHY DIET

- Fresh ingredients that do not have an unpleasant odor due to rancidity
- Whole foods such as whole ground grains, not "flours," "mill runs," or "by-products"
- Concentrated protein sources known as "meal" (as in "lamb meal" or "beef meal") are preferred over whole meats (listed only as "lamb"). This is not to be confused with "by-product meal."

"Meal" simply refers to the process of removing up to eighty percent, but no less than forty-five percent, of the ingredient's water content. There is more *meat protein* for your money, since water only adds to the weight of the ingredients. Weight is listed on the product label by the heaviest to lightest ingredient. It is very deceiving to find chicken (or turkey, rabbit, fish, and other animal sources) listed first, when the majority of protein is coming from grains, not animal protein. The cost of the product is considerably less when a protein other than an animal protein is used. One pound of meal is equal to approximately three pounds of whole meat, and since there is an additional charge to dehydrate meat , many companies use the meat to draw you to the label, but use a cheaper ingredient for the actual protein—a protein source that could trigger allergies.

Look for identifiable and digestible animal protein or fat sources such as beef, beef meal, lamb, lamb meal, lamb fat, chicken, chicken meal or chicken fats, turkey, ostrich, etc., not vague terms like "meats," "mammal," or "animal fats."

Look for USDA Grade A or B animal protein sources, preferably raised without growth hormones or recently given antibiotics (possible with some free-range raised lamb, cattle, or chicken).

USDA Grade 1 or 2 whole grains, preferably free of chemical pesticides or herbicides. Organic grains are not yet cost-effective for use in commercial pet foods (if your pet's food claims "organic," demand written certification), but "pesticide-free" is available or "washed" grains are possible. Beans are an excellent source of protein as well. If you are cooking for your pet at home, buy the best you can afford!

Balanced, combined proteins and grain sources suit most pets better than single-source ingredients, contrary to popular belief. Vegetable and fruit fiber should be present, such as carrots and apples, for proper digestion, natural flavoring, and trace nutrients. Fiber is important to elimination, and is full of nutrients when additionally provided in whole grains. Quality sources of fat are necessary for energy and good coats. Vegetable or fish oils should be used, rather than animal fats. Because cats have a higher metabolism than dogs, they need the higher fat content, and high-quality animal fats are acceptable.

Price. Often, the cheaper foods are actually more expensive, meal to meal, because you have to feed so much more than a better-quality diet with less filler.

Product should be fresh when purchased. Check the manufacture date, not the expiration date. Manufacturers will never admit the food won't really last a year. Never feed your pet food, especially naturally preserved food, that is older than six months, unless it has a completely sealed, airtight, barrier bag. Stale food not only doesn't taste good, it has lost most of its nutritional value through oxidation, and the ingredients are no longer as bio-available.

INGREDIENTS TO AVOID IN A HEALTHY DIET

Foul-smelling ingredients should be avoided at all cost. No matter what the date is on the bag, smell it when you open the bag and if it smells rancid, don't feed it to your pet.

Greasy food. If you see oil on the bag or on the cans of pet food, it is high in animal fats or tallow. These can include rendered carcasses and recycled cooking grease from restaurants. These fats are difficult to digest and are often rancid prior to the manufacturing process.

Animal by-products such as "beef by-product," "lamb by-product," "chicken by-product" are a mixture of the whole carcass including feces, cancerous tumors, hide, hooves, beaks, feathers, and fur. "Meat" or "meat by-products" are a mixture of whatever mammals, including road kill, rats, and other dogs and cats that got ground up together. "Poultry by-products" are a mixture of whatever feathered animals, including pigeons, got ground up together, and should definitely not be fed to your pet.

Grain by-products such as "mill runs," "flours," "middlings," "husks," and "parts" should be avoided at all costs. They lack nutritional value because all the nutritional value has been removed. They may be harsh on an animal's digestive and eliminatory tracts, and irritate the body as it attempts to process them. These cheap fillers are used as additional protein sources to increase the finished product's weight and mass, although they are non-digestible and therefore cannot be assimilated.

Fillers such as powdered "cellulose" and "cellulose fiber" can include recycled newspaper, sawdust, and cardboard. "Plant cellulose" is usually ground peanut hulls—which are very damaging to sensitive colon tissues. Beet pulp or grain by-products have no significant nutritional value, but do add bulk and weight to the finished product.

Yeast is a cheap source of B vitamins, amino acids, and some nutrients. Touted for flea control and a shiny coat, yeast can contribute to allergies by burdening the liver and interfering in proper digestion.

Sugar is added to most commercial diets and treats. Known as "sucrose," "beet pulp," "molasses," "cane syrup," "fruit solids," and of course, "sugar," it is a very cheap, heavy filler (cost effective for the manufacturer) and is also addictive (the pet will want more of the same). Additional sugar in the diet is the primary trigger of weight problems, diabetic conditions, and behavioral problems in pets.

Symptom Reversal

Once you have established a good foundation by detoxification and proper diet so that the body can draw strength to fuel its curative process, it is time to address the individual needs of your pet. Although the basic curative process is the same for all living beings, each one of us has our own unique journey toward symptom reversal.

All of our symptoms have a history, unique to our own experiences. A youthful body can cope with a multitude of stresses and maintain some balance, but as the body grows older and becomes more burdened as its biological processes begin to slow down naturally, it becomes overwhelmed by a stressful lifestyle.

The history of disease and the curative process is determined by the age of the pet, how genetically compromised they are, the quality of their lifestyle, and the severity and duration of the symptoms. I have never seen an animal that was too old, too weak, too young, too sick, or too hopeless to respond to holistic animal care. Is every case a complete success? That depends on your definition of success. Every animal's symptoms, when addressed holistically, experience some positive change.

Seventy-five percent of pets respond immediately to detoxification and nutritional support, and a large number experience long-term symptom reversal. Fifteen percent need additional naturopathic (including acupuncture or acupressure, chiropractic, and massage), plus homeopathic and/or herbal support, to complete the curative process and effectively reverse their allergies.

Eight percent of pets might need some medical or chemical support: short-term symptom suppression through antihistamines or antibiotics (when symptoms are severely damaging to the pet's overall health) and steroids (when lack of curative response is life-threatening). Many of these animals can benefit from short-term support until the natural support they are receiving takes over. Unfortunately, probably half of these animals were given chemicals because the body's attempts to rebalance were misunderstood. Classic symptoms of detoxification were visible, but the owner or veterinarian arrested the process with medical treatment. Some of these owners later returned to detoxification successfully, but others remained in the cycle of symptom suppression for years before they allowed the detoxification process to be completed. Others simply gave up.

Two percent of suffering pets will always have allergies regardless of what is done. Symptoms can be suppressed holistically and/or chemically for short-term relief, but as soon as treatment is stopped, the cycle begins anew. These pets are either too genetically compromised or too overwhelmed by their condition to ever successfully reverse their dis-ease on their own. Remember that the more holistic the lifestyle, the easier it will be to keep the pet's resistance to toxins high and their biological functions processing to their fullest potential—even if you choose to use medication as well. Each year your pet lives a holistic lifestyle, its body will continue to strengthen, and many symptoms will become easier to handle, or even reverse themselves later on. Detoxification also protects the liver, kidneys, and other vital organs from toxic drug side effects.

Zaezar, my fourteen-year-old female Rottweiler, has a genetic predisposition to respiratory allergies. Because she was raised on natural diets and looked so healthy, I had become lax in her supplement regimen. She then developed symptoms around five years ago, and her breathing was so compromised at times that we were forced to use over-the-counter antihistamines, which made her stare off and lose her appetite. We addressed her immune weaknesses holistically, and this year she needed fewer doses of her herbal antihistamine—she is so much stronger! She again is enjoying life and is a prime example of the fact that even in older, genetically compromised pets, through adhering to a holistic lifestyle and supporting symptoms overall—even if temporary suppression is needed—positive change can occur.

Common sense is the most valuable tool you possess for reversing allergic symptoms. Ask yourself if what you are doing is getting you the results you want. If not, re-evaluate, but do continue addressing the problem. Not doing something is *not* an option. *Nothing comes from nothing.* On countless occasions, people exclaim, "I thought I'd just wait and see if it got any better on its own." They are shocked that the condition gets worse! By the time they get around to doing something, it may be too late, the body may be too weakened, or the dis-ease too deep, and it is so much harder to regain balance!

The only time that it is appropriate to do nothing is during detoxification or a curative response, where the health of the animal may temporarily become worse as the body attempts to rebalance itself. To do something (to suppress symptoms) during this time only stops the curative process, and drives the imbalance deeper into the body.

It is appropriate to address symptoms through holistic animal care when:

- Any non-life-threatening symptom has been present for four to eight hours, and the body is slow to respond.
- There are acute (sudden) symptoms from overexertion or toxins: rashes, pustules, digestive upset, discharges, stiffness, irritability or emotional stress, including withdrawal (often the result of exhaustion due to excessive scratching or pain).

- There are acute flare-ups of chronic (ongoing) symptoms, especially during detoxification.
- Known triggers are present, such as during high-exposure days. Many of my allergic symptom reversal suggestions can also be applied as a preventative.
- A curative response has been ongoing for more than forty-eight hours, and the body needs relief.

It is appropriate to address symptoms through allopathic, veterinary care when:

- There is any life-threatening acute symptom, especially paralysis, respiratory difficulties resulting in hyper-panting, an excessive heart rate present for two to four hours, loss of consciousness, excessive dehydration, or uncontrollable shaking.
- High fever is present for more than twenty-four hours.
- Chronic symptom aggravation for more than twenty-four hours results in loss of mobility, uncontrollable digestive upsets, urinary dysfunction, or other severe symptoms.
- Unmanageable infectious states, *even if mild*, have lasted for four to six weeks.

When in doubt, seek out a trusted professional to support your pet's process.

Helpful Hints

Feed a high-quality diet and supplement at least twice per day—more often if needed to help stabilize blood sugar, support the immune system, and reduce the allergic reaction.

Supplement with the proper nutrients, including glandular products and herbs, for a strong foundation from which to stimulate the body's curative response.

Utilize homeopathy to help maximize the body's curative potential, especially the processes of detoxification and symptom reversal.

Use synergistic modalities such as chiropractic care, massage, touch and energy therapies, including giving acupressure therapy at home in-between veterinary acupuncture sessions. Home therapy will prolong the benefits received in a clinical visit.

Maintain a holistic animal care lifestyle, even in-between reactions, to help enhance the body's defenses and further balance the body's weaknesses. With each month the body will continue to gain balance and strength, including joint support and resistance to general sensitivities. Remember, symptom suppression—even holistically *but* without constitutional support—only leads to a reoccurrence of symptoms, not a long-term reversal of dis-ease.

Do not underestimate the power of nature; recognize that nature can take longer to suppress a symptom than a drug, but often will do the job more completely.

Support the curative power of nature and avoid interfering with it. Use chemicals and medications carefully. Avoid vaccinations whenever possible.

Use common sense. Address changes in your animal's health or behavior as soon as possible, and pay attention to what your pet's symptoms are telling you. For example, if your dog's skin irritation increases the day after you bathe him, don't continue to use the same shampoo or to bathe him so frequently.

Don't sabotage the healing process by incorrectly utilizing diets, veterinarian-prescribed medications, or natural supplement products. Read the directions. Ask questions! The more you know and understand, the more successful you will be.

Remember, it can take three to six weeks for detoxification and increased assimilation of nutrients to begin establishing the necessary foundation for a successful curative process. During this time old cells are being replaced with newer, healthier cells, which will bring change to the overall condition. Therefore, it is best to allow the body some time to respond on its own before adding too many other ingredients to the mix. Provide a high-quality multiple vitamin and mineral supplement with basic herbal or homeopathic support for the first month or two, until you better understand the specific underlying imbalance. Remember that close to eight out of ten pets successfully reverse their allergies with this alone. Additional supplements or medications may overwhelm the body with ingredients it doesn't need and may interfere with the body's natural curative process. Explore each product available to see what they specifically recommend in your situation. Be sure to read ingredient labels carefully, and follow all instructions listed on any products you choose to use on your animals.

Homeopathy is safe to use in addition to herbs or medications, although allopathic drugs may interfere with a homeopathic remedy's potential to trigger the curative process. Utilize homeopathy to its fullest potential by following a few simple suggestions, as it is very helpful in reducing acute flare-ups and supports symptom reversal on a deeper level than herbs or supplements alone. Homeopathy can often be the key to reversing a deeper acute or chronic weakness. Although a lot of emphasis is placed on potencies, I have found many remedies to be successful in a wide range of potencies, so I'm more inclined to support getting whatever potency is available to you, whether it is a 6X and not a 3C. For the majority of acute reactions, even if due to chronic conditions, utilizing the lower potencies will effect change. These potencies range anywhere from 3X to 30C. For long-term reversal of a specific disorder, utilizing the higher 200C potency will be effective, after lower potencies have brought the acute reaction under control. High potencies, such as Ms, should be used with professional guidance. By giving the body a boost with homeopathic remedies, other supplements will act more quickly and effectively.

When beginning a homeopathic remedy, I recommend building up its action in the body through frequent dosing. You cannot overdose your pet. Give one dose orally, according to the manufacturer's recommendations, every fifteen minutes for the first hour, then every hour until there is relief. To maintain relief, dose a minimum of twice daily for an additional one to two weeks. More frequent dosing may be administered as needed. Resume homeopathic treatment or any another appropriate remedy whenever the symptom presents itself, and follow this schedule until there is complete reversal. Long-term maintenance is also possible through a weekly dose of the most beneficial remedy.

I prefer liquid remedies because they are easier to administer. If the dropper touches your hands or your pet, rinse it off before returning it to the bottle. Most remedies come in sugar pellets (use as is) or tablets (crush inside a piece of paper first for best application). To avoid contamination and a reduction in efficacy, do not handle these remedies with your bare hands. Rather, use the cap or a clean piece of paper to administer the dose. Always allow at least fifteen minutes between food or strong extracts when giving homeopathic remedies.

Symptoms: A to Z

This chapter lists the most common symptoms associated with allergies, as well as some that are not generally associated with allergies, but which I suspect are related. Your pet may be experiencing a slightly different symptom than what I describe. Please try to match your particular needs as closely as possible to one of the symptoms listed.

Abscesses can erupt, especially around the chest and back. This occurs most often during a curative response or detoxification process. As one of its defenses against toxins, the body will pocket an irritating substance or allergen (sometimes for years) to keep it from establishing a deeper hold. Detoxification releases these toxins from the fatty tissue where they are stored and releases them into the bloodstream for elimination. Since the skin is the largest eliminatory organ, abscesses may occur. At the first sign of swelling and accompanying heat, a dose of homeopathic *Belladonna* or *Sulphur* may discourage the full formation of an abscess.

Whether you suspect a foreign object or not, use the homeopathic remedy *Silica*, which encourages eruption and drainage. Since the abscess itself is actually a foreign object, *Silica* will generally work well. If not, try *Mercurius*, especially if thick pus has formed and the surrounding skin has become angrier. Apply a warm, damp cloth to the area for fifteen minutes at a time to encourage eruption of the abscess. This will also soothe your pet. Homeopathic *Hepar Sulphuricum* is the best remedy for abscesses too painful to touch, and it can be used in conjunction with the Silica.

Once there is drainage, be sure to keep the area clean and dry. It is helpful to trim away a little fur around the site to expose it to more air. This encourages healing and makes it easier to treat the abscess topically. Clean it with a solution of fifty percent hydrogen peroxide and fifty percent water, then apply a little *Tea Tree* or *Calendula lotion* to help encourage healing and prevent worse infections. Treat topically at least once a day, twice a day if the abscess is large and angry. (See Infections.)

Adrenal Malfunction is common in animals who are also exhibiting allergic reactions, especially those with chronic skin conditions. Often, it can actually be caused by previous cycles of steroid treatments which are commonly used to suppress allergy-related symptoms. You may want to recommend a book to your veterinarian entitled *Pet Allergies: Remedies for an Epidemic*, by Alfred J. Plechner, DVM, and Martin Zucker.

Testing for hormonal or cortisol levels will benefit you, no matter what you decide to do. If nothing has seemed to work, utilize any medication that is appropriate for you and your animal. Pets who have not responded well to natural modalities are often diagnosed with deeper glandular malfunctions, which, when addressed, help stimulate the curative process.

There are many wonderful, natural glandular products available. I prefer *glandulars in powder or tablet form* to homeopathic ones, but do not disregard a homeopathic remedy combined with a potentized glandular *in addition* to a tableted form. Homeopathic glandulars work on a deeper level and are beneficial to overall support, whereas tableted glandulars actually feed the gland directly, providing more substantial support in reversing glandular weakness. *Multi-glandulars*, a combination of several glands, are beneficial in supporting the weaker gland, but make sure that the combination contains sufficient amounts of the particular gland you need to stimulate and support. Add another single glandular product to the multiple, if needed. (See Cushing's Disease.)

Allergy Reactions in general can be successfully suppressed with a few doses of homeopathic remedies in lower potencies (3X to 30C). Give one dose orally, according to the manufacturer's recommendations, every fifteen minutes for the first hour, then every hour until there is relief. Always allow at least fifteen minutes apart from food or strong extracts. When in doubt, treat the most obvious symptom first, then focus on any specific ones that manifest later.

Homeopathic Remedies for Allergic Reactions

- *Arsenicum* is used for general irritations, hot spots, digestive imbalances, or toxicity-related symptoms such as reactive arthritis.
- *Sulphur* is used for a wide variety of skin conditions associated with intense itching which becomes worse at night in warm surroundings. Scratching may seem to satisfy the pet temporarily, but often will result in increased itching and burning. *Sulphur* is also good for greasy skin.
- *Apis* is good for intensely itchy skin that is aggravated by warmth, including the warmth the body may give off when covered in rashes. The skin is noticeably red.
- *Rhus Tox* is helpful when the animal is rubbing or scratching its skin, when the animal gets wet, or when cold weather seems to aggravate itchy skin. It is especially good for irritations around the head.
- *Urtica Urens* addresses extensive eruptions, hives, or welts that are very itchy. Usually the skin is dry and aggravated by warmth or bathing. (These conditions are non-responsive to *Apis* or *Sulphur*.) It is also good for profuse discharges from mucous membranes. Symptoms may be localized to the right side of the body.

- *Sabadilla* is a popular hay-fever remedy, addressing common upper-respiratory symptoms such as asthma, spasmodic sneezing, watery nasal discharge, facial itching, irritated ears, and red, runny eyes.
- *Euphrasia* is another excellent remedy for allergy-related eye and tear duct irritations.
- *Nux Vomica* addresses the majority of digestive imbalances, including gas, vomiting, diarrhea, or lack of appetite, especially when dosed with *Arsenicum*.

Herbal antihistamines and anti-inflammatory products are very effective and a good alternative to over-the-counter drugs such as *Benadryl* or veterinary prescriptions such as *Prednisone*. I highly recommend that you use a combination of homeopathic remedies for acute reactions and herbs to lessen sensitivity, which may reduce a more severe reaction.

Herbs for Allergic Reactions

- *Yucca Root* has been used for centuries by indigenous cultures to reduce general inflammation. Current studies have confirmed that bio-available steroidal saponins (found mostly in pure extract form, rather than the fibrous powder that is a waste product of extraction) perform as effectively as their chemical counterparts (steroids such as *Prednisone*), without the serious drug side effects. *Yucca* enhances the action of other, more specific-use herbs, by supporting liver function and detoxification.
- *Chinese Ephedra* is a powerful antihistamine which quickly reduces inflammation. This herb has been abused as a stimulant, but it is very safe when used as directed. *Ephedra* reduces the itching of a histamine reaction and can be used for both topical (eyes, ears, skin) and internal (irritable bowels, inflamed respiratory passages) symptoms.
- *Marshmallow and/or Bayberry Root* reduces inflammation in general, and is helpful with detoxification of histamines and in reducing respiratory stress.

- *Eyebright Herb* helps address general allergy symptoms affecting the eyes.
- *Stinging Nettle Leaf* reduces general redness and irritation of the skin, eyes, and ears. It can also help reduce irritation of the anal glands and inflamed joints.
- *Red Clover Blossoms* are useful in reversing skin eruptions, as well as reducing coughs and bronchitis. This herb supports immune function.
- *Eyebright, Bayberry Root Bark, Golden Seal Root, Calamus, and Stinging Nettle Leaf* act together to contract swollen mucous membranes associated with hay fever and allergies. Their anti-bacterial properties help keep infections of the eyes, ears, and respiratory system in check.
- *Turmeric Root, Black Catechu, Grindelia Floral Buds, and Lobelia,* combined, protect the liver from circulating antigens and allergens, thereby reducing infections and skin or intestinal irritations associated with airborne, urea, and food-related allergies. This combination supports the adrenal glands when epinephrine is needed by the body during inflammatory responses generated by allergens. It also is indicated for all disorders of hypersensitivity, including allergies, asthma, dermatitis, irritable bowel syndrome, reactive arthritis, and food-related digestive disorders.
- *Red Clover Blossoms, Stinging Nettle Leaf, Cleavers Herb, Yellow Dock Root, Burdock Root, Yarrow Flowers, Plantain Leaf and Corm, Licorice Root, and Prickly Ash Bark* purify the blood and drain excess lymphatic fluids. This combination improves metabolism by carrying more blood and nutrients to the cells, thereby promoting greater excretion at the cellular level. It is useful for eczema, psoriasis, tumors, cysts, acne, and other skin disorders such as mange. It is also helpful for lymphatic edema and toxemia, including reactive joint inflammation.

Nutritional Supplements for Allergic Pets

- Vitamin C (1000 mg. per twenty-five pounds of body weight per day) helps strengthen the bodyís resistance and curative response. Works as an infection fighter and antihistamine.

- Vitamin A (2500 IU per twenty-five pounds of body weight per day) with Beta Carotene (1200 IU per day)and Vitamin E (50 IU of d-Alpha) to stimulate the immune system and tissue rejuvenation.
- Vitamin B-Complex (50 mg. to 100 mg. per day regardless of size, as smaller pets utilize it faster) provides essential vitamins needed to protect the body from allergens and facilitate a curative response by relieving stress.
- Antioxidants such as Selenium, Super Oxide Desmutase and Garlic help eliminate toxins that lower the petís resistance to allergens.
- Omega-3 and Omega-6 Fatty Acids help reduce the itch of dry skin while promoting tissue repair. Supplements are helpful until nutrients can balance the bodyís ability to assimilate fatty acids better.
- MSM is a sulfur-based nutrient, which helps reduce tissue inflammation, and promotes improved skin elasticity and coat condition.
- Minerals such as Zinc (5 mg. per twenty-five pounds per day), Chromium (5 mcg. per twenty-five pounds) and others support tissue repair and build resistance.
  (See Symptoms: A to Z; Immune System Dysfunction, for support with the more severe allergy symptoms.)

Anal Glands can become impacted in pets, especially dogs, who have been fed poor-quality diets and whose digestive and eliminatory systems do not function properly. This creates irritation and itching around the anus, and the pets will scoot their rear ends across the floor and chew at them, eventually infecting the area.

If the pet owner squeezes or drains these glands incorrectly, it will only damage them further, making them even more susceptible to impacting. Please have these glands professionally expressed by a veterinarian, no more than every six weeks at first, then tapering off until you can go yearly if necessary.

You can encourage drainage of these glands by holding a compress, soaked in a warm solution of six ounces pure water, two ounces *Witch Hazel*, with twenty drops of *Calendula Extract*, ten drops of *Golden Seal Extract*, and ten drops of *Yucca Extract*. Rinse well with a fresh solution, followed by a topical application of *Calendula*, *Tea Tree Oil*, and/or *Aloe Gel*. Keep some topical solution in the refrigerator; it will feel especially soothing on irritated and inflamed tissues. Soak a cotton pad and hold it gently against the area for a few minutes, or spray it on as needed. Repeat two to three times a day until swelling and redness is gone.

Apply *Vitamin E* and/or *Jojoba Oil* directly to tough or scarred tissue to soften it. Avoid petroleum-based products, which will further irritate the area and encourage bacterial infection. Such products can become poisonous if ingested frequently.

A few doses of homeopathic *Apis* or *Hypericum* for irritation and *Arsenicum* or *Nux Vomica* for detoxification can greatly reduce discomfort. *Hepar Sulph* can help reverse infected glands. It is more effective when combined with *Arsenicum* or *Nux Vomica* and an herbal antibiotic such as *garlic*, *Echinacea* or *Golden Seal*.

Dried *Chinese mushrooms*, such as *Shiitake* and *Reishi*, are very healing to anal gland tissues, and together with other fiber-producing ingredients (apple pectin, guar gum, psyllium) can help stimulate a complete evacuation of stool from the colon, which will reduce toxic waste from backing up the anal glands. *Astragalus Root* is useful for prolapsed conditions of the anus and impacted anal glands. It works as a diuretic to flush wastes, reduce edema, and promote the discharge of pus. *Garlic* is also indicated. Don't forget flower remedies, such as *Mimulus*, or a *Rescue* combination, if your pet refuses to allow you near without a fight. (See Abscesses, Infections.)

Anemia is a common symptom in allergy-suffering pets. I believe that many cases of anemia associated with allergies are the result of liver complications. Common side effects of allergy-related anemia include lack of stamina, a depressed appetite, poor coat condition with slow tissue repair, poor immune function, muscle weakness, pale-colored gums, and dull eyes. Sometimes the faint odor of metal is present on the breath. More serious anemia needs proper diagnosis and treatment, but borderline anemia is commonly reversed with proper nutrition.

Allergy-related anemia is the body's inability to produce more red blood cells to counteract the liver discarding its cells when this valuable organ becomes burdened and begins malfunctioning. Iron supplementation is a well-known treatment for anemia, and will quickly reverse symptoms. Always use a good-quality source such as an *iron proteinate*, iron chelated with an amino acid, for superior absorption. Be careful not to overdo iron supplementation, as it can easily become toxic. The first symptom of toxicity is constipation. Limit daily levels to around 10 mg. for cats and small dogs, and 20 mg. for medium to large dogs. In addition, provide *chromium* to aid in iron assimilation, which reduces the body's need for higher levels of iron. I also utilize *Alfalfa*, both in herbal (nutrient-rich) or lower-potency homeopathic form. *Taraxacum* is also a good homeopathic choice, as is its herbal twin, *Dandelion*.

Although liver is a popular remedy for anemia, avoid feeding it to your pet on a regular basis. Liver is a primary detoxifying organ and stores excess toxins it has eliminated from the blood. When you feed this organ to your pet, you are also feeding it concentrated toxins, including growth hormones and antibiotics.

Appetite Problems, especially loss of appetite, can occur during curative responses to dis-ease or drug toxicity. First, however, be sure there is no fever present, and that your pet is not dehydrated. (See Fever and Infection.) Also determine the level of stress your pet may be experiencing and address that, as stress can also interfere with appetite. (See Behavioral Problems.)

For nutritional support, feed up to 100 mg. of B-Complex vitamins per day regardless of body weight. This, in addition to a short fast, can quickly stimulate the appetite. Often, a lack of appetite is the result of a toxic overload.

Try a few doses of homeopathic *Arsenicum* for general appetite loss; *Nux Vomica* when appetite loss is accompanied by one or more symptoms including nausea, vomiting, stool problems, flatulence; or *Belladonna* for mostly nausea, empty retching, and vomiting as well as an aversion to drinking. A dose or two daily, *especially fifteen minutes prior to feeding*, can also help to stimulate appetite. Several flower essences, especially *Mimulus, Star of Bethlehem*, and *Rock Rose*, or a combination, can often settle an animal enough so that it begins to regain an appetite.

Arthritis can flare up in conjunction with, or as a direct reaction to, certain allergy conditions, especially those involving congested or malfunctioning liver, kidneys, adrenal, and thyroid glands. Symptoms can best be suppressed and possibly eventually reversed homeopathically and/or herbally, while the physical structure (joints, ligaments, muscles, and tendons) is strengthened through nutritional supplementation.

Homeopathic Remedies for Reactive Arthritis

• *Arsenicum* is an excellent general homeopathic arthritic remedy.

- *Arnica* reduces swelling, general muscular pain, and discomfort.
- *Bryonia* helps when the pet is stiff upon standing and cannot walk out of it.
- *Rhus Tox* is for the pet that is stiff upon standing but can walk out of it.
- *Hypericum* reduces nerve irritation and pain found in animals who are constantly licking their legs and feet, and sometimes even their backs.
- *Ruta* is best for severe tendon or ligament strains, common in nutritionally depleted pets. Combine with *Hypericum* for degenerative intervertebral disc disease.

Herbal Remedies for Reactive Arthritis

- *Yucca* is a very effective anti-inflammatory. The stalk and roots contain steroidal saponins, which react in the body similar to chemical steroids, but without the side effects that chemical steroids produce. Saponins also reduce tissue inflammation and pain. Be sure to use a cold-pressed *Yucca* extract, rather than powder or tincture. The extract contains up to eighty-five percent more bio-available saponins and is easier on the digestive tract than other forms.
- *Garlic* is a wonderful supplement for joints affected by allergy reactions.
- *Milk Thistle, Licorice, Alfalfa, and Dandelion* are all excellent herbs for liver and blood detoxification, reducing free radicals that can irritate joints.

Nutritional Supplements for Arthritic Pets

- *Vitamin C* (1000 mg. per twenty-five pounds of body weight per day) helps strengthen ligaments and tendons, reduce inflammation, and lessen allergy sensitivities.
- *MSM* is a sulfur-based product which not only helps to reduce inflammation, but is also wonderful for poor skin and coat conditions.
- *Glucosamines* help replenish synovial fluid, a shortage of which can create the rubbing of bone upon bone, resulting

in pain and encouraging calcium build-up, which can result in more severe arthritis.

- *Boron* aids proper calcium absorption and strengthens bone density. It also helps the body avoid calcium build-up or over-calcification, common in arthritic conditions.

Asthma (See Upper Respiratory Problems.)

Behavioral Problems are often associated with allergy symptoms. Discomfort can trigger aggression, though some animals respond with nervousness, shyness, or complete withdrawal. Flower essences and homeopathic remedies work really well at addressing the underlying emotional aspect of most behavioral problems.

Flower Essences and Homeopathic Remedies for Behavioral Problems

- *Star of Bethlehem* is good for learned stresses. For example, if you yelled at your cat for licking her coat when she was in her bed, she may not settle down when you are ready to go to bed yourself.
- *Mimulus* is the remedy for minimizing fears of all types: fear of the bath, fear of having ears or eyes cleaned, fear of wind, storms, etc.
- *Rock Rose* is used for present terror.
- *Vine* is for the overbearing pet.
- *Impatiens* quiets the pet that is always impatient and always a little nervous, despite your reassurance.
- *Aconite* addresses behavior that is the result of situations which produced sudden shock or fear.
- *Ignatia* helps to reduce symptoms related to grief or loss.

Unfortunately, nervousness, fear, or any intense emotion can reduce immune function and leave a pet very susceptible to allergens. Herbs such as *Valerian Root*, *Hops Flowers*, *Skullcap*, *Chamomile*, and *St. John's Wort* (which also helps balance hormones) help to relax the pet, allowing them to rest more comfortably and sleep more deeply—all necessary for supporting the curative process.

Bladder and Kidney Problems sometimes occur in conjunction with allergy conditions, especially during the elimination of waste products, including allergens. The deeper stages of detoxification can also produce the very symptoms more commonly related to bladder or kidney problems, such as difficulty when urinating or incontinence, discharges or infectious states (WBC and bacteria seen in urine sample), and metallic-smelling urine. Once detoxification is complete, these symptoms suddenly clear up on their own. Avoid using antibiotics to treat any minor infections during this time. Give the body at least four to six weeks of holistic support to reverse infections on its own. (See Detoxification and Infections.)

Nutritional and Herbal Supplements for Bladder and Kidney Problems

- Increase *Vitamin C* to at least 1000 mg. per day per twenty-five pounds of body weight to acidify the urine, kill off bacteria, and support tissue repair.
- *Provide plenty of fresh pure drinking water* and monitor daily water intake. Add water to food to increase fluid intake, if needed.
- Utilize herbal extracts such as *Juniper Berry, Uva Ursi, Usnea Lichen, Plantain* and *Buchu Leaves*, and *Horsetail Grass* for increased urine output and to dissolve blockages.
- *Plantain Leaf and Corm, Buchu Leaves, Corn Silk, Horsetail Grass, Arnica Flowers,* and *Thuja Leaf* work well to control incontinence, by regulating and strengthening the musculature and toning the membranes of the urinary system.
- *Usnea Lichen, Uva Ursi Leaf, Pipsissewa Herb, Echinacea Angustifolia* and *Purpurea Roots, Flowers, and Seeds* are very

fast-acting, powerful antibiotics for urinary tract infections, including cystitis and nephritis. They contain certain therapeutic agents that are known to target the very bacteria that creates the irritation and inflammation. These herbs are safer for long-term treatment and crisis care in older or more debilitated pets, and can be used safely with prescribed antibiotics. While drugs attack the acute infection, these herbs increase the pet's natural resistance. When the pet is weaned from the chronic drug use, the herbal properties will take over the task of protecting the urinary tract and reducing the likelihood of infection reoccurrence.

- *Yucca Extract* can relieve inflammation and pain in the urinary tract.

Homeopathic Remedies for Bladder and Kidney Problems

- *Cantharis*, the most popular remedy for bladder and kidney problems, is used for pets with a frequent, strong urge to urinate, possibly with pain. When painful elimination is interfering with output, it can help to stimulate flow of urine. It is also beneficial in reversing incontinence due to bladder irritation.

- *Apis* provides great relief to those who experience similar bladder and kidney symptoms (urgency to urinate, urinary pain, bladder irritation, etc.). Symptoms include much straining to pass only a few drops of urine, an abdomen that is sensitive to touch, and a bleak attitude.

- *Mercurius* is indicated for a small volume of dark urine, often present with infection. Urination is often painful at the beginning of flow, with uncontrollable urges.

- *Berberis* is helpful with obvious back pain from urination or motion.

- *Sarsaparilla* addresses even the most severe pain, especially when accompanied by dribbles of urine.

- *Gelsemium* supports control of urine flow, especially when incontinence is due to partial paralysis of the bladder. The urine is often profuse, clear, and watery.

- *Belladonna* is another excellent remedy for incontinence due to acute urinary infections, or when high levels of phosphates are present in urine. The urine is almost continually being released by the body and can be dark and cloudy.

Serious problems during urinating, such as excessive straining with little or no urine output for twelve hours or more, should be evaluated immediately by a veterinarian.

Cancer can often be the end result of a long-term bout with allergies, as an "allergic" condition will often accompany the other distressing symptoms of cancer. Cancerous cells take so much energy from the body that it will become very susceptible to allergens. Unfortunately, I have seen many immune system problems, including Feline Leukemia, Feline Infectious Peritonitis (FIP), Tick Fever, Valley Fever, and chronic anemia (a possible pre-cancerous state), in pets originally diagnosed and treated chemically for "allergies" or chronic skin, ear, and eye problems. I believe that the constant stress upon the body, due to allergy reactions themselves—as well as the chemicals and drugs used to treat them—weakens the animal's constitution and their curative potential, and encourages damaged cells to mutate into cancerous cells.

Many of the allergy relief recommendations in this book are applicable to the treatment of cancerous conditions. In both cases, the underlying imbalance is likely to be in the immune system, and allergies or cancer are the symptom. (See Immune Dysfunction.)

Cataracts occur in a large number of pets who suffer season after season from allergy problems (not necessarily only in the eyes), and chemical treatment for these problems. Cataracts are a direct result of irritants and toxins from environmental and dietary sources that damage sensitive eye lens tissues, causing them to cloud over. A lack of nutrients such as *Vitamin A*, *E*, and *Zinc* (often depleted during allergies) can also encourage the formation of cataracts. Along with proper nutrition, I have successfully reversed cataracts with homeopathic *Silica 200C* daily for four weeks, then *Silica 1M* weekly for four weeks, then *Silica 10M* weekly for four more weeks. These higher doses of Silica should be used under the supervision of an experienced practitioner.

Chewing can drive both the pet and the owner nuts. It seems as if it will never end. It is potentially very harmful to your pet. The constant stress of chewing and licking quickly leads to emotional and physical exhaustion, further weakening the immune system. Treat these more as a nervous habit rather than a symptom. Obviously, you need to first rule out any rashes, abrasions, cuts, flea or tick bites, etc., that may be triggering the chewing and address them topically. (See Allergy Reactions.)

Then utilize herbal and/or homeopathic remedies for irritability and nervousness. You will be amazed at how effective these are, even if you do not believe that your pet has any emotional issues. Flower essences work well also.

Herbal Remedies for Chewing

* *St. John's Wort* helps balance hormones and brain chemistry to provide a sense of well-being and calmness. It also acts as a sedative and facilitates pain relief.
* *Skullcap* supports the nervous system and helps control seizures that can accompany severe allergic reactions.
* *Chamomile* is an effective calmer and works well, especially for digestive allergies possibly triggered by anxiety.
* *Wild Oats* is an excellent nerve tonic and helps rebalance the nervous system while it decreases itching.
* *Valerian Root* is another well-known calming and restorative herb.

Homeopathic Remedies for Chewing

- *Aconite* addresses chewing resulting from situations associated with sudden shock or fear and increased anxiety.
- *Ignatia* helps to reduce chewing related to grief or loss.
- *Arsenicum* can reverse an irritable disposition.

Flower Essences for Chewing

- *Rock Rose*, *Chicory*, and *Holly* are beneficial for chewing.

Colitis and Irritable Bowel Syndrome are common symptoms associated with allergies, especially food allergies. However, constant stress of other allergy conditions can also result in diarrhea, constipation (or alternating between the two), mucuos-covered stools, flatulence, and even slight blood in the stool. *Nux Vomica* and *Arsenicum* are a good homeopathic combination to use initially. Digestive enzymes can also be appropriate, but I recommend that you limit their use to a few weeks at a time. The overuse of enzymes can imbalance digestion further. Calming herbs, especially *Wild Oats* and *St. John's Wort*, are also helpful. Fiber supplementation with whole grains, fruits, and vegetables can provide proper bowel care and encourage evacuation. *Yucca* is a wonderfully soothing herb, as are *Aloe* and *Slippery Elm Bark*. (See Constipation and Diarrhea.)

Constipation is a common symptom associated with allergies. Whereas diarrhea is often associated with food allergies, alternating constipation and diarrhea, or constipation alone, can also occur because of allergies. Constipation can weaken the body because the waste products have not been properly eliminated and toxins will be reabsorbed from the colon into the bloodstream. Several factors can contribute to constipation, including medications such as antibiotics and antihistamines, which are often used for allergies.

First eliminate any possible culprits:

- hard-to-digest pet food ingredients, such as "plant cellulose" (often soy castings, peanut shells, or husks of any kind that are used as filler/fiber in pet food)
- lack of exercise, when an animal has been confined for six hours or more and not able to relieve itself when needed
- inadequate fluid intake
- excessive ingestion of fur or hair, due to licking and chewing
- ingestion of non-digestible objects such as rocks, rubber, bone, or feathers
- poor sources of dietary fiber

Psyllium seed or husks are commonly used to regulate bowel movement, but, when used alone, often can be too harsh on the digestive tract. Combine psyllium with other fruits and vegetables such as *carrots, apple fiber* and *pectin, guar gum* (a misunderstood, but excellent, source of natural fiber that swells to retain water), and *bran. Chinese mushrooms*, such as *Shiitake* and *Reishi*, which are also high in fiber, can help to reverse chronic colon conditions, including pre-cancerous growths. Cooked *oatmeal*, added to meals or given alone with vegetable, fish, or meat broth, not only is high in fiber, but also has detoxifying properties to help eliminate old fecal material from the bowels. (See Digestive Disorders.)

Corneal Ulcers often occur in pets that have suffered from inhaled, ingested, or environmental allergies. Lack of tears, scratching and rubbing of the eyes, as well as nutritional deficiencies, contribute to the development of ulcers on the outer protective layer of the eyeball.

Once your veterinarian has diagnosed this problem, it can often be quickly reversed with twice-daily applications of natural *Vitamin E* (d-Alpha, not dL-Alpha) directly to the inner eyelid, so blinking can spread it over the entire eye. This can be a little sticky, but it will not interfere with your pet's eyesight. It will help reverse inflammation and irritation and prevent permanent damage. Use a 200 IU capsule, applying half in the morning and the other half at night. Apply a high-quality, natural tear solution as well, when needed, to prevent drying of the eyes that may occur due to reduced tear production or tear duct blockage.

Feed additional *Vitamin E*, 100 IUs per day for cats and small dogs, up to 200 IUs for larger dogs. Use a good-quality daily multiple vitamin and mineral supplement that includes at least 5,000 IU of *Vitamin A* for cats and small dogs, or 10,000 IU for larger dogs.

Herbs such as *Eyebright*, *Golden Seal*, and *Calendula* tinctures can be used separately or in combination. Dilute one drop tincture to one ounce of filtered or distilled water. These herbs can help fight infection, unblock the tear duct, and soothe the eyes when applied as an eye wash prior to applying the Vitamin E. (See Eye Problems.)

Cushing's Disease is a serious malfunction of the adrenal gland, requiring a veterinarian's help. Many veterinarians have reported that when holistically addressing the adrenal malfunction associated with allergies, symptoms of Cushing's Disease have also improved.

Symptoms can include fatigue, hair color loss or poor coat growth, excessive shedding, slow tissue repair, and a droopy belly. The skin may be gray and leathery, resembling an elephant's skin. Within six months of natural support, this skin condition, which is generally believed to be irreversible, may actually be reduced in severity by up to eighty percent. (See Adrenal Malfunction.)

Cystitis (See Bladder and Kidney Problems.)

Demodectic Mange (See Skin Parasites.)

Dental Problems are often overlooked and shouldn't be. They will weaken the body's defenses against allergens. It is vital that you keep your pet's teeth and gums clean and free of infection. Daily brushing with a wet washcloth and a little natural toothpaste (avoid fluoride whenever possible) can work wonders in a short time. If heavy tartar has developed, it can be safely scraped away with a dental tool made for pets.

Unless it is life-threatening or teeth need to be removed and pus pockets drained, avoid anesthesia, which can further weaken your pet's immune system. Instead, use a homeopathic *"Rescue" Flower Remedy* or *Aconite* to calm the pet if needed, and proceed to clean the teeth as best as you can.

Some practitioners will clean your pet's teeth without anesthesia, so seek them out if needed. Also consult with your veterinarian if you ever suspect a serious infection or find loose or broken teeth. (See Infections.)

Dermatitis. Skin problems are a very common manifestation in pets suffering from allergies. Flea bites are also a common source of dermatitis. When the skin becomes irritated, inflamed, and itchy, pets begin to scratch, rub, chew, and lick themselves. The skin then becomes so irritated and inflamed that other problems arise: hair loss, dandruff, greasy skin, pimples, and hot spots.

A *hot spot* is an irritated, open area of skin caused by scratching or biting, which can result in infection. Keep the area dry and clean. Clip away the hair around the hot spot to make it easier to clean and treat topically. If a pet has chronic dermatitis and has been exposed to many cycles of antibiotics, a staphylococcal infection may arise that is difficult to treat.

Avoid the use of coal tar-based or chemically medicated shampoos. Do not bathe too often; when the skin is severely irritated, bathe no more than every two to four weeks. Spot cleaning and disinfecting can be done whenever needed. Over-frequent whole body bathing can actually worsen the condition by drying out the skin, thereby encouraging greasy skin. (Body oils will try to replenish themselves quickly and heavily to counter such drying.) Instead, spot clean and disinfect the skin whenever needed.

Feed potent doses of a high-quality *garlic* supplement (500 mg. to 1000 mg. per day for small dogs and cats, up to 2000 mg. for medium- to large-sized dogs). In addition, *Vitamin C* and other nutritional support for allergies will do more to clear up hot spots permanently than topical treatment alone. (See Infections, Skin and Coat Problems.)

Diabetes is another disease frequently associated with a history of allergy-related problems. I believe that there is a strong relationship between blood sugar stabilization (or lack of it) and allergy sensitivities. Many pets suffering from allergies finally responded to medical treatment for their allergy symptoms when, later in life, they were diagnosed with diabetes, and their blood sugar was stabilized through insulin and diet.

When allergies present themselves early in your pet's life, adhere to a holistic animal care lifestyle to help prevent a diabetic condition from developing. Feeding at least twice per day, or three to four smaller meals per day, as needed during allergy-prone times, can also help to reduce stress and to support the body's resistance to allergens.

Herbal support, in addition to proper diet and supplementation, can help reduce the amount of insulin needed. *Devil's Club Root and Bark, Indian Jambul Seed, Dandelion Leaf and Root, Uva Ursi Leaf,* and *Turmeric Root* can eliminate the need for insulin in many pets. This formula strengthens the pancreas, promoting better production and utilization of insulin, and also normalizes and restores the organs and glands associated with carbohydrate and sugar metabolism. Re-synthesis of glycogen promotes greater balance of glucose and is indicated in both hyper- and hypoglycemia.

Diarrhea is often associated with food allergies, although I have seen it manifested in pets suffering from other allergy stresses, especially constant scratching and biting—all that nervous energy just churns up the bowel. *Psyllium seed or husk* is the most commonly used fiber to help regulate bowel movement, but often it can be too harsh on the digestive tract when used alone. I highly recommend combining it with other fruit and vegetable fiber sources such as *carrots, apple fiber and pectin, guar gum* (a misunderstood, but excellent, source of natural fiber that swells to retain water), and *bran.*

Chinese mushrooms, such as *Shiitake* and *Reishi,* have long been noted for their fiber content as well as their curative potential in reversing chronic colon conditions, including pre-cancerous growths (which may be irritated and triggering the diarrhea).

Cooked *oatmeal,* added to meals or given alone with vegetable, fish, or meat broth, is not only an excellent source of fiber, but also has detoxifying properties and can help eliminate old fecal material from the bowels. Old fecal material can become toxic (especially with bacterial infection) and can trigger the body's attempt to eliminate the irritation, resulting in the diarrhea.

Add to the oatmeal a high-quality *garlic* supplement (500 mg. to 1000 mg. per day for small dogs and cats, and up to 2000 mg. for medium- to large-sized dogs). This regimen will give your pet natural antibiotic support.

These homeopathic remedies are effective in relieving diarrhea and associated symptoms. Use *Arsenicum* for general symptoms, *China* for debilitating fluid loss, and *Nux Vomica* for vomiting and/or appetite loss.

Herbally, use *Yucca* and/or *Calendula Extract*, *Liquid Chlorophyll*, and *Slippery Elm Extract or Powder* to soothe irritated intestinal tissues. Be sure that fluid intake is maintained, as diarrhea can quickly dehydrate your pet. Add one-half teaspoon of *raw honey* per twenty pounds of body weight per day to fluids or herbal preparations. Honey is not only soothing to an irritated colon, it is antiseptic, and it provides energy for a weakened pet. (See Digestive Disorders.)

Digestive Disorders are very common during grass and pollen allergy season, and most are associated with food and other environmental allergies. The second most common complaint I hear (skin problems is number one) is lack of appetite, vomiting, stool changes, or hair balls. The use of digestive enzymes can be beneficial in the short term, but you will have to address the actual imbalance for long-term symptom reversal. (See How to Reverse Your Pet's Allergies Holistically.)

Homeopathy is very effective in reversing acute stomachaches, liver inflammation, stool changes, and the underlying stress that often accompanies these digestive disorders.

Homeopathic Remedies for Digestive Disorders

- *Arsenicum* is used for general digestive imbalances or toxicity and will alleviate most allergy-related digestive disorders, especially if there is liver or spleen involvement, or if the disorder has been triggered by a season of one dose per month of flea and tick control products.

- *Nux Vomica* also addresses the majority of digestive imbalances, including gas, vomiting, lack of appetite, or stool problems (especially alternating between constipation and diarrhea). It complements *Arsenicum*.

- *Carbo Veg* is helpful when the pet is overweight, has chronic stool problems, seems to have trouble digesting well, and burps soon after eating. This remedy is extremely beneficial when used with *Nux Vomica*, and is a good senior pet tonic.

- *Belladonna* is for the sudden onset of gastrointestinal symptoms. After initial use, it should be tapered off slowly and then followed by a more specific remedy. *Belladonna* is also indicated for acute colic and pancreatic imbalances resulting in a "fatty" stool.

- *Urtica Urens* addresses a lack of appetite often accompanied by extensive itchy eruptions, hives, or serious welts. These afflictions, which are not responsive to *Apis* or *Sulphur*, often appear in conjunction with digestive or eliminatory problems, as well as dry skin aggravated by warmth or bathing. Digestive problems may also be associated with profuse discharges from mucous membranes, ears, and eyes. Symptoms may be localized to the right side of the body.

- *Phosphorus* is indicated if the digestive problems include great debilitation, fluid loss, or frequent vomiting or diarrhea soon after meals. *Phosphorus* quickly eliminates blood (from old fecal material, viral or bacterial detoxification) or fatty mucus (from pancreatic imbalance) in the stool.

- *Podophyllum* can be used when profuse, offensive-smelling stools occur. Stool color may be yellowish or greenish, is often completely liquid, or begins formed and turns loose as the bowel movement progresses, and can also be accompanied by dry heaves or gagging.

- *Pulsatilla* aids diarrhea or mucous-covered stools, which are often greenish in color. This stool will frequently change in character or color, even during the bowel movement. Diarrhea is likely to be worse at night or aggravated by warmth. Symptoms, such as nausea, vomiting, or diarrhea, are not too severe. Food is often the culprit, especially if it is high in animal fats or rancid ingredients. The offending food might be vomited up partially digested. The tongue may become coated with a thick white or yellowish material.

- *Ipecac* can quickly subdue vomiting, especially when it is related to food or ingested chemical allergies.
- *Colocynthis* is indicated for pets who are cramping or whose stomachs are rumbling. There may be other symptoms. They want to lie on a hard surface, or they will respond positively when you rub their belly. Movement, drinking, or eating will aggravate symptoms.
- *Bryonia* addresses those pets who are also cramping or whose stomachs rumble, but they avoid hard surfaces or respond in pain when their stomachs are rubbed. They may also exhibit arthritic pains as a result of an allergic reaction.
- *Mercurius* benefits pets who have marked upper digestive tract and liver involvement, especially when they feel pain when they are touched or lying on the right side. Stools may be whitish-gray or yellowish green. Often, pets are very irritable with swollen gums that bleed easily, and their tongues may be slightly swollen and coated with a yeast-like substance.
- *Lycopodium* is another excellent liver remedy, especially with back pain, gas, bloating, discomfort, and rumbling of the stomach soon after meals. These pets seem to fill up quickly after only a few bites of solid food.
- *China* supports pets that have chronic liver involvement with digestive imbalances who are very sensitive to touch and open air. They chill easily and seek to hide, especially after meals. Although they may crave cold water, it will cause them to burp up partially digested food.

Herbal remedies can support reversal of many symptoms associated with digestive disorders, can increase digestion or assimilation, and can stabilize appetite. Many pets cannot tolerate herbs on an empty stomach. In fact, the herbs themselves may create some of the digestive stress. When pets have digestive upsets, it is best to give herbs with a little food, until they are better tolerated, or you might try to obtain better-quality herbs.

Herbal Remedies for Digestive Disorders

- *Yucca Extract* provides natural steroidal saponins, which effectively reduce inflammation within the digestive system, including the stomach and intestinal lining as well as the liver, gallbladder, spleen, and pancreas. A reduction in excessive peristalsis (a squeezing response of the intestines, to process and move digested material toward the colon) can help to relieve diarrhea due to allergic and inflammatory responses. Intestinal pockets, ulcerations, and inflamed intestinal valves that block passages (often associated with allergy-related colitis) have also responded well to *Yucca* supplementation.

- *Garlic* is excellent for digestive complaints. Not only is it antiseptic and a natural antibiotic, it effectively supports proper digestion and colon health through its anti-parasitic and anti-yeast properties. Higher allicin contents are beneficial in reversing general diarrhea, flatulence, and fatty stool deposits.

- *Peppermint Leaf* or *Fenugreek Seed* helps to reduce intestinal gas, cramping, and colic, prevents fatty deposits, repairs digestive tissue ulcerations, and fights infection.

- *Dandelion Leaf* is an excellent tonic for the liver and gallbladder.

- *Siberian Ginseng Root* stimulates resistance against food or reactive allergies.

- *Milk Thistle Seed* supports proper liver function and detoxification.

- *Calendula Extract* contains therapeutic components that soothe sensitive and irritated digestive tissues, including the stomach and intestinal lining, as well as the liver, gallbladder, spleen, and pancreas.

- *Devil's Club Root Bark*, *Indian Jambul Seed*, *Dandelion Leaf and Root*, *Uva Ursi Leaf*, and *Turmeric Root* reduce the occurrence of soft, fatty, off-colored stools. (See Diabetes.)

- *Cascara Sagrada Bark*, *Barberry Root*, *Senna Leaves*, *Rhubarb Root*, and *Cayenne* clean out the intestinal tract. A detoxified colon is fundamental to rebalancing the digestive system and increasing assimilation of nutrients necessary for proper health. These herbs can also prevent or reverse parasitic infestation.

- *Fennel Seed*, *Ginger Root*, and *Anise Seed* relieve gas, cramping, and mucus while stimulating proper digestion and peristalsis.
- *Shiitake* and *Reishi Mushrooms* have been used by the Chinese for centuries to prevent and treat cancers associated with the digestive system. Colon cancer in particular responds well to their incredible healing properties. A dramatic reduction in food sensitivities is often the result of long-term supplementation. (See Appetite Problems, Constipation, Colitis, Diarrhea.)

Ear Mites (See Skin Parasites.)

Ear Problems commonly occur in allergy-sensitive pets. The liver, a primary organ affected by allergens or toxins, has a relationship to the ears and eyes. As the liver becomes burdened, the ears begin to exhibit symptoms associated with allergy problems, becoming more prone to irritation from grasses, pollen, and molds, as well as from foods and chemicals.

Allergies often occur during warmer weather when dogs especially bathe and swim more. Water may become trapped in the ear channel, encouraging bacteria and yeast to grow there, leading to an ear infection. Foxtails and other foreign bodies may also become lodged in the ear. Always check first to see if you can find anything in the ear and remove it prior to treatment. If needed, seek proper removal by a veterinarian.

Ears can be effectively cleaned with a home-made solution of two ounces distilled or purified water, one teaspoon of *Witch Hazel*, one teaspoon of white vinegar, and six drops of *Calendula Extract*. Add an additional six drops of *Golden*

Seal Extract if infection is suspected. Use a cotton ball to squeeze a little of this solution into the ear. Rub the outer base of the ear to massage the solution into any debris that needs to be removed (you may hear a slight suction-like noise inside the ear). Allow your pet to shake out their ears, then wipe out the rest of debris and fluid with a soft tissue wrapped around your finger. To avoid damage, do not insert anything down into the inner ear, but rather let the tissue absorb any impurities. Follow cleanings with an application of *Calendula Extract, Aloe Gel,* or *Vitamin E.* Use *Hypericum, Calendula,* or *Arnica Cream* around the flap and opening, if pain is present.

Be careful not to use heavy, oil-based ingredients or vegetable oils, unless you are attempting to dissolve a foreign body or kill ear mites (see Skin Parasites). Although such oils may seem to be conditioning the ear and reduce irritation, they may also nurture a bacterial or yeast infection, by providing a warm, moist, oxygen-free environment. For dogs with ear flaps in the down position, tie them up over the head with an elastic hair band to encourage air circulation. As little as one hour of air circulation per day can reduce bacterial or yeast growth, and encourage healing.

To dissolve a suspected foreign body which is not creating severe pain or bleeding, warm up two tablespoons of *garlic-flavored cooking oil* (which will help discourage bacterial growth), or use soybean oil and add a capsule of *garlic extract* to it, plus six drops each of *Golden Seal* and *Mullein Extract,* and 200 IUs of *Vitamin E.* Drip it down into the ear with an eye dropper, spoon, or cotton ball. Keep it in the ear for as long as your pet will tolerate it, and massage the base of the ear to loosen the object further before flushing the ear out with the cleaning solution. Repeat several times per day until the object is dislodged, usually within a day or two. This will dissolve hardened debris as well as many plant particles. Never force fluid into the ear with pressure, or you may drive the object further in, making it harder to remove it safely yourself.

Grapefruit Extract ear drops can also be applied after cleaning the ear to fight bacterial and yeast infections. *Mullein and Garlic Oil* ear drops are also excellent for irritated and infected ears.

Avoid alcohol-based products, which can irritate the ears further—unless you suspect water is trapped in the ear canal, in which case a few drops of pure alcohol can dry up the fluid residue. Don't worry about the alcohol found in herbal extracts—very little alcohol remains by the final dilution. Avoid glycerin-based herbal extracts in general, unless your pet has a sensitivity to alcohol. I have found them to be less therapeutically potent than alcohol-based products.

Proper grooming is also beneficial for keeping the ears free of infection or waxy build-up. Many breeds, such as Poodles, Terriers, and Cocker Spaniels, grow hair close around the ear, and sometimes even in it. You must pull the hair from in the ear and clip the outer areas short, to help air circulate. Many dog breeds who are prone to ear infections have a closed flap ear rather than a standing flap ear. A standing ear flap allows additional air to circulate, drying ears quickly and thoroughly, thus avoiding infection.

Herbal Remedies for Ear Problems

- *Garlic* is vital to eliminating ear problems. Use a high-potency supplement for basic antibacterial support. Because it is high in natural sulfur, garlic helps heal irritated tissue and reverse eruptions and irritations.
- *Yucca Extract* works as well as steroids, reducing inflammatory responses. (See Allergic Reactions.)

- *Spilanthes Flowering Tops and Roots, Oregon Grape Root,* and *Myrrh Gum* work well together for more serious yeast and/or fungal infections.
- *Red Clover Blossoms, Stinging Nettle Leaf,* and *Cleavers* help soothe irritated tissue, often seen in severely itchy ears with rashes or tiny pimples inside and around the ear.
- *Turmeric Root, Black Catechu, Grindelia Floral Buds,* and *Lobelia* is a combination that protects the liver from circulating antigens and allergens, thereby reducing ear infections and irritations associated with airborne and food-related allergies. Ear problems, particularly those accompanied by digestive disorders, respond well to this combination.
- *Eyebright, Bayberry Root, Calamus Root, Golden Seal Root,* and *Stinging Nettle Leaf* is an excellent combination for ear infections directly related to grass or pollen sensitivities, which are often accompanied by eye irritation or discharge. Symptoms include very itchy, blotchy, infected ear tissue, often visibly swollen.
- *Echinacea, Red Root, Baptisia Root, Thuja Leaf,* and *Prickly Ash Bark* clean the blood and lymphatic systems, and activate the body's immune response. This combination is beneficial when the ear condition is associated with autoimmune dysfunction, which is chronic and difficult to address. Other symptoms that respond well to this combination include ear flap hematoma or blood blisters, which are often the result of trauma due to scratching.
- *Sheep Sorrel, Burdock Root, Slippery Elm,* and *Turkey Rhubarb Root* are often the key to chronic symptom reversal.

Homeopathic remedies can quickly reverse acute symptoms associated with ear-related allergies.

Homeopathic Remedies for Ear Problems

- *Arsenicum* and *Apis* combined are effective for sensitivities to airborne allergens, especially itchy ears.
- *Silica* and *Arnica* combined are effective when a hematoma (large blood blister) has formed on the ear flap. The *Silica* expels the blister, while the *Arnica* helps heal it pain-free. (See Abscesses.)

- *Graphites* works well for foul-smelling discharge.
- *Hepar Sulph* helps control sensitive, inflamed ears with discharge.
- *Mercurius* relieves boils and hematoma found on the external ear canal, and is good for reversing thick, yellow discharge that is often foul-smelling and bloody.
- *Rhus Tox* is indicated in chronic ear infections. It works well with *Arsenicum*.
- *Hypericum* can be used if ears are extremely sensitive to touch.
- *Aconite* supports the pet who has become overly sensitive about being petted on the head during or after being treated for ear infections.

If the ear seems more irritated, begins to bleed profusely, becomes unbearably painful, or develops a severe discharge, and is non-responsive to home treatment within a few days, then seek out veterinarian care immediately. Do not take ear problems lightly, as chronic inflammation and infections can lead to permanent damage, resulting in deafness. Reliance on a chemically based, medicated ear wash or drops can also permanently damage the sensitive tissues of the ear. (See Infections, Skin and Coat Problems, and Skin Parasites.)

Eczema (See Skin and Coat Problems.)

Emotional Problems (See Behavioral Problems.)

Eye Problems are almost always involved in allergy responses and often accompany ear symptoms, as both the eyes and ears are indicative of liver function. Allergens and antigens can overwhelm the liver. Resistance to airborne sensitivities, in particular, is compromised. Check your pet's eyes daily, and wipe away any matter present. Always address eye problems quickly, as chronic irritation or infection can permanently damage the eye, possibly leading to cataract formation and even blindness.

To clean away slight discharge, use a warm, damp cotton cloth. Always use distilled water on the cloth. Wipe in the direction of the eyelashes to avoid further irritating the eye. Start in the inside corner, allow your pet to close the eye before gently wiping lightly downwards towards the outside corner.

To remove heavy matter or copious discharge, in and around the eye, use a warm, wet cotton pad or ultra-soft cotton paper towel. Hold it gently against the eye, allowing it time to soften any hardened matter. Gently wipe the inside of the lid to remove discharge on the eyeball, being careful not to introduce any dirt or crust into the eye. Then remove the remaining matter on the outside lashes. Repeat as often as needed. Do not allow the eye to remain crusted-over and shut. This will encourage infection and can damage the eye or tear duct permanently.

Follow cleaning with an application of natural eye drops made by diluting six drops of *Calendula Extract* in a couple of ounces of distilled water. For very irritated or dry eyes, apply a few drops of natural *Vitamin E oil*, every other day, directly to the inside of the lower eyelid. Be careful not to scratch the eye. Blinking will disperse the Vitamin E. A few drops of *Golden Seal Extract* can also be added to eye drops, if infection is present (See Infections.) This will also help to open up tear ducts, and encourage natural lubrication. (See Infections.)

Herbal Remedies for Eye Problems

Always supplement with herbs to strengthen and cleanse the eye, increase resistance to allergens and infections, and support anti-inflammatory and antihistamine action. Proper nutritional and herbal supplementation can prevent and even reverse cataracts, a common side effect of chronic eye irritation.

- *Yucca Extract* works as well as steroids in reducing inflammatory responses (See Allergic Reactions.)

- *Chinese Ephedra, Mullein Leaves*, and *Lobelia* is a natural antihistamine combination, which quickly reduces acute responses that result in itchy eyes and tearing. It is an excellent, short-term symptom suppressor, allowing other herbs and nutrients a chance to build up the body.

- *Eyebright, Bayberry Root, Calamus Root, Golden Seal Root*, and *Stinging Nettle Leaf* address symptoms that include very itchy, dry eyes, often visibly swollen, or weepy with infection.

- *Red Clover Blossoms, Stinging Nettle Leaf*, and *Cleavers* soothe irritated tissue, which can manifest as severely inflamed, itchy eyes, with rashes or tiny pimples around the eyes, face, and ears. These herbs can help prevent and eliminate tiny eyelid cysts, and are excellent for mange-reactive eye sensitivities.

- *Echinacea, Red Root, Baptisia Root, Thuja Leaf*, and *Blue Flag Root* clean the blood and lymphatic systems, and activate the body's immune response. This combination is beneficial when the eye condition may be associated with autoimmune dysfunction and can be difficult to address. Other symptoms that respond well to this combination include tiny blood blisters, or cysts around the lids, often the result of trauma due to scratching.

- *Sheep Sorrel, Burdock Root, Slippery Elm*, and *Turkey Rhubarb Root* can be the key to chronic symptom reversal. (See Immune System Dysfunction.)

Homeopathic Remedies for Eye Problems

- *Arsenicum* and *Apis* is a great combination for sensitivities to airborne allergens, especially itchy, runny eyes.

- *Silica* and *Hypericum* work together to help unblock tear ducts. Also follow directions for abscesses, if needed.

- *Euphrasia* encourages tearing to reduce dryness and irritability.
- *Aconite* is beneficial when the eyes are severely inflamed and red, with hard, swollen lids. Eyes seem aggravated by wind and sunlight, and tend to tear profusely.
- *Pulsatilla* is indicated for creamy, profuse eye discharges.
- *Hypericum* and *Arnica* should be used if there is injury and pain, due to scratching or heavy rubbing of the eyes. (See Corneal Ulcers.)

Fatty Tumors (See Skin and Coat Problems.)

F.U.S. or Feline Urological Syndrome is often seen in cats with chronic allergies, especially after months of chemical therapies (steroids, antibiotics, and even pest control products). As the body attempts to eliminate these toxins, the urinary tract can become irritated and even blocked with bacteria or mineral crystallization. Detoxification can often clear up this chronic condition, but additional support may be needed.

Herbal Remedies for F.U.S.

Herbal care can strengthen and tone the bladder and kidneys, encourage urine output and elimination of blockages and infection.

- *Juniper Berry*, *Spring Horsetail*, *Corn Silk*, and *Goldenrod Leaf* will stimulate proper urine production and elimination, reduce obstruction and stone formation, and soothe irritated membranes. Their disinfecting properties help reduce infection.
- *Usnea Lichen*, *Uva Ursi Leaf*, *Pipsissewa Herb*, *Echinacea Angustifolia* and *Purpurea Roots*, *Flowers, and Seeds* act as a natural antibiotic. (See Bladder and Kidney Problems.)
- *Yucca* acts as a general anti-inflammatory and an alternative to steroids. (See Allergic Reactions.)

Homeopathic Remedies for Acute Symptoms of F.U.S.

- *Cantharis* or *Aconite* reduce irritation and pain during urination.
- *Arsenicum* is indicated for chronic urinary blockages. (See Bladder and Kidney Problems.)

Fleas (See Skin Parasites.)

Fleabite Dermatitis (See Skin and Coat Problems.)

Hair Loss (See Skin and Coat Problems.)

Heart Problems, such as a rapid heartbeat, can accompany chronic allergy reactions, which stress this organ due to powerful surges of histamine and adrenaline. Excessive panting can mistakenly be attributed to allergies, yet it can possibly indicate a more serious heart condition, so be sure to report any changes in breathing patterns or weakness with exercise to your veterinarian.

Homeopathic Remedies for Heart Problems

If heart problems are primarily affected by allergic reactions, then homeopathic remedies should quickly address them.

- *Aconite* is beneficial when labored breathing and tumultuous heart action follow allergic response, or when heart inflammation is suspected.
- *Arsenicum* is indicated when weakness is triggered by a chemical reaction, particularly by vaccination, topical skin treatment, or pest control products. The heart may fluctuate between rapid and labored beating.
- *Iberis* helps regulate an irregular heartbeat and reduce palpitations.

Hot Spots (See Skin and Coat Problems.)

Immune System Dysfunction is often at the root of allergy conditions. It is vital that you address and support proper immune function. Unfortunately, it is common to see pets develop more serious dis-ease, such as cancer, after struggling for years with allergy-related symptoms. Many people have also reported an increase or sudden development of allergies after the pet has been treated medically for another condition, such as kidney problems. In each case, the underlying weakness is the immune system, and the best way to reverse most symptoms is to strengthen the immune system first.

Vitamins C, A, B-Complex, and *E* cannot be surpassed for their immune-enhancing capabilities. Several other vitamins, minerals (such as *Zinc, Selenium*, and *Chromium*), and amino acids can enhance the efficacy of these nutrients, so a properly balanced and therapeutically potent multiple supplement is essential.

In addition, several herbal and homeopathic remedies support resistance to antigens or infections, reduce catabolic waste (responsible for many skin and digestive symptoms), and eliminate damaged or mutated cells, which are often responsible for a weakened immune response and the genesis of cancerous cells.

Herbal Remedies for Immune Dysfunction

Herbal extracts, preferably organic and standardized (which have a stronger guaranteed potency) should be diluted in purified water, tuna water, or apple juice and given on an empty stomach for optimum therapeutic response. If your pet is suffering from digestive disorders, herbs may be better tolerated when given with meals.

- *Sheep Sorrel, Burdock Root, Slippery Elm*, and *Turkey Rhubarb Root* is an old indigenous herbal remedy to eliminate catabolic waste and stimulate the immune system. Chronic cases often need this foundation for detoxification and increased resistance. Several dog breeds, such as Dalmatians, Cockers, and German Shepherds, and cat breeds such as Siamese or Persian, who genetically suffer chronic immune weaknesses, often fail to recover until this combination is introduced. This combination is a good preventative herbal remedy.

- *Echinacea* and *Golden Seal Root* are nature's antibiotics. They are effective in fighting off viral, bacterial, yeast, and fungal infections while stimulating the immune system in general. These natural antibiotics cleanse the blood, lymph system, liver, and kidneys. They can be used topically for the reversal of abscesses, gangrene, and pus discharge, and also to open up blocked tear ducts. Use in addition to garlic.

- *Astragalus Root* helps tone and stimulate the spleen, an important immune system organ. It fights infection, helps restore appetite, and reduces fatigue and diarrhea resulting from infection. It is also useful for prolapsed conditions of the anus and impacted anal glands. It acts as a diuretic to flush wastes, reduce edema, and discharge pus, and it increases metabolism and aids the adrenals.

- *Pau d'Arco* is beneficial for the whole body. It stimulates the immune system, heals wounds, combats infections, kills viruses, and is effective against cancers (including lupus and leukemia), cysts, and tumors. Use it both internally and topically for ringworm, hot spots, eczema, psoriasis, and staphylococcal infections. It provides excellent general support and can reverse cystitis, colitis, gastritis, diabetes, liver and kidney weaknesses. *Pau d'Arco* relieves arthritic pain and is easier for very sick, weakened, or older pets to tolerate than *Golden Seal Root*.

- *Lomatium Root*, *Echinacea Root*, *Spilanthes*, *Chinese Schizandra Berry*, and *Licorice Root* promotes strong anti-viral activity and have immune-enhancing properties. This combination of herbs enhances cellular immunity and liver function to protect healthy cells from antigens and viral infection. They are indicated in cases of chronic viral infections that have not responded well to medications, or where the liver may be inflamed. They can be used with *Astragalus* for debilitating or chronic infection.

- *Echinacea, Red Root, Baptisia Root, Thuja Leaf*, and *Prickly Ash Bark* acts as blood and lymphatic drainers, while activating the body's immune response. Symptoms that respond well to this combination include: conditions associated with autoimmune breakdown and catabolic waste build-up, tiny blood blisters, pimples/feline acne, skin ulcerations, lymphatic engorgement, chronic infection, tumor growth, cysts, fluid cysts, cancer, reactive arthritis, and wasting disease.
- *Spilanthes Leaf and Root, Grape Root, Juniper Berry, Usnea Lichen*, and *Myrrh Gum* combined are very powerful anti-fungal and anti-yeast agents. This combination is beneficial in reducing Valley Fever spore infestation. It helps the immune system respond to yeast overgrowth, vaginal infection, penis discharge, and ringworm.

Homeopathic Remedies for Immune Dysfunction

Homeopathic remedies can facilitate the immune system's response to a specific toxin, allergen, bacteria, virus, yeast infection, or parasitic infestation, although they should never be relied upon solely to address immune imbalance. If an animal is severely debilitated, you may have no choice but to use a homeopathic remedy along with nutritional and herbal supplementation to facilitate a currative process.

- *Arsenicum* quickly triggers detoxification and elimination through the liver and kidneys, and stimulates other vital organs and glands responsible for proper immune response. *Arsenicum* prepares the body to utilize immune-enhancing nutrients.
- *Gelsemium* is an outstanding remedy for the first signs of disease, especially fever. Use this remedy for pets who seem very needy and want to be held when they begin to feel poorly, or have had a relapse after a long, debilitating illness and weak recovery.
- *Echinacea* is good for reoccurring boils, intolerance of insect bites, and lymphatic engorgement. It helps address fatigue often experienced during immune problems.

- *Sweet Chestnut* is a flower remedy that addresses deep despair and anguish often experienced by a pet after a long illness.

Infections can be addressed through herbal extracts, preferably organic and standardized (stronger, guaranteed potency). These should be diluted in purified water or apple juice and given on an empty stomach for optimum therapeutic response. If your pet is suffering from digestive disorders, then herbs may be better tolerated when given with meals. If this is the case, then increase the dose slightly to help assimilation.

Herbal Remedies for Infections

- *Sheep Sorrel, Burdock Root, Slippery Elm*, and *Turkey Rhubarb Root* is an indigenous herbal remedy for pets suffering from chronic or severe infections. Genetically or medically compromised animals need this foundation for detoxification of catabolic waste and increased resistance to re-infection. (See Immune Dysfunction.)
- *Echinacea* and *Golden Seal Root* (See Immune Dysfunction.)
- *Astragalus Root* aids the adrenals, to support the body while it burns up infections. (See Immune Dysfunction.)
- *Pau d'Arco* kills viruses and helps reduce fever. It provides excellent general support and can reverse weakness from chronic infection and long-term medication. (See Immune Dysfunction.)
- *Lomatium Root, Echinacea Root, Spilanthes, Chinese Schizandra Berry*, and *Licorice Root* promotes strong anti-viral activity. (See Immune Dysfunction.)
- *Echinacea, Red Root, Baptisia Root, Thuja Leaf*, and *Prickly Ash Bark* act as blood and lymphatic drainers, while activating the body's immune response to fight infection. (See Immune Dysfunction.)
- *Spilanthes Leaf and Root, Grape Root, Juniper Berry, Usnea Lichen*, and *Myrrh Gum* combined are very powerful anti-fungal and anti-yeast agents. (See Immune Dysfunction.)

Homeopathic support has never been, in my opinion, very effective in fighting infection by itself, but should be used instead to address acute secondary symptoms. (See Abscesses, Immune System, Skin and Coat.)

I.B.S. (Irritable Bowel Syndrome) (See Colitis.)

Lick Granuloma can develop on the body, especially around the lower legs and feet, after chronic trauma through licking has occurred. A hard knot slowly develops that is often the primary spot for a pet's focus. Therefore, it is commonly thought to be simply obsessive behavior, and the condition is not addressed until the granuloma appears. Once the licking has become chronic, it has also become obsessive behavior and is not addressed during treatment. Although the "allergy" itself has been suppressed, compulsive licking of the area will help continue the symptom cycle by re-irritating the skin. Although surgical removal of the granuloma is often the suggested course of veterinary treatment, I discourage it because it can return with a vengeance and is then more likely to become cancerous.

Licking is a serious concern for many pet owners. Excessive licking is not only irritating to the owner, it will quickly exhaust the pet. The pet's vital healing energy is redirected to address this fatigue, instead of supporting tissue repair and immune stimulation.

Although normal daily self-grooming includes licking the body clean, obsessive and chronic licking can lead to hair balls (see Digestive Disorders), skin eruptions (see Skin and Coat Problems, Allergic Reactions), even growths (see Lick Granuloma). Homeopathic *Arsenicum* works the best for constant licking, especially when a build-up of urea is involved. *St. John's Wort* and *Chamomile* help reduce the anxiety often associated with excessive licking. Try Flower Essences, such as *Rescue* or *Mimulus*, which are good for obsessive behavior. (See Abscesses, Allergy Reactions, Chewing, Digestive Disorders.)

Liver Problems are often at the root of allergy-related symptoms. The liver can become additionally burdened and congested by yeast or chemical allergy-relief products. Immediately eliminate all yeast from your pet's diet, supplements, treats, or pest control products if you suspect liver disorder.

The liver is a primary organ of the digestive, eliminatory, and immune systems. All these systems are involved in the proper functioning of the body's defenses against allergens and its tissue repair capabilities. If you are to be successful in reversing your pet's condition, you will have to be truly concerned about the care and support of your pet's liver.

Herbal Remedies for Liver Problems

* *Yucca* and *Garlic Extract* are wonderful detoxifiers of the liver. They help to reduce general inflammation and organ congestion. (See Allergic Reactions.)
* *Milk Thistle Seed, Yellow Dock Root, Burdock Root, Echinacea Root, Sarsaparilla Root,* and *Oregon Grape Root* work together to promote optimum liver health and function. These herbs address improper fat and fatty acid metabolism, detoxify the liver and blood, reduce bacterial and hormonal disorders associated with poor liver function, and alleviate chronic skin conditions.
* *Lomatium Root, Echinacea Root, Spilanthes, Chinese Schizandra Berry,* and *Licorice Root* target cellular immunity and liver function to protect healthy cells from antigens and viral infection. (See Immune System Dysfunction.)

- *Echinacea*, *Red Root*, *Baptisia Root*, *Thuja Leaf*, and *Prickly Ash Bark* act as blood and lymphatic cleansers, reducing liver toxicity. (See Immune System Dysfunction.)
- *Sheep Sorrel*, *Burdock Root*, *Slippery Elm*, and *Turkey Rhubarb Root* is an old indigenous herbal remedy for catabolic waste elimination and liver stimulation. (See Immune System Dysfunction, Anemia, Digestive Disorders.)

Mange (See Skin Parasites.)

Mites (See Skin Parasites.)

Nose Discharges (See Upper Respiratory Problems.)

Obesity (See Weight Problems.)

Pancreatitis (See Digestive Disorders.)

Paralysis or muscular weakness can result from a reaction to an allergen, such as yeast, pollen, food by-products, chemicals, or medication. After proper veterinarian diagnosis to rule out a bacterial, viral, or neurological origin, nutritional, herbal, and homeopathic remedies can reduce inflammation, pain, and debility. Often a proper course of holistic treatment can result in complete reversal of allergy-related paralysis.

Homeopathic *Arsenicum*, given in frequent dosages, will provide initial relief of many symptoms. *Hypericum* is indicated when nerve involvement is suspected. Taper off to two daily doses, until recovery is complete.

Yucca, in the standardized extract form only, is as effective as steroids in most applications. If needed, *Yucca* can even be used in conjunction with steroids to reduce the need for heavy doses of this potentially harmful medication, until the herb alone can be used for long-term maintenance. (See Allergic Reactions, Arthritis.)

Pregnancy is mentioned here because many pets first develop allergy-related symptoms while pregnant. This is understandable, given the amount of toxins produced by supporting the growing litter. Some pets never have a reoccurrence of allergic reactions, although it is more common to find that pregnancy was the genesis of chronic allergies for many animals. Please do not breed any pets which have a history of immune-related conditions such as allergies, or you probably will pass on this genetic weakness.

Research carefully any herbal supplements you use during pregnancy, since many herbs can be dangerous for both mother and babies.

Herbs to Avoid During Pregnancy

- *Angelica, Golden Seal, Pennyroyal* can cause uterine contractions.
- *Mugwort, Wormwood, Rue* also stimulate contractions.
- *Barberry, Cascara Sagrada* can be too strong of a laxative during pregnancy.
- *Buchu, Juniper Berry*, because it is a strong diuretic, and is too dehydrating.
- *Ephedra (Ma Huang)* is too strong of an antihistamine to use during pregnancy, although when it is used as a tea, it may help respiration without stress.

If you suspect that your pet is currently pregnant, and exhibits allergy symptoms, use the alternative fasting program and a well-balanced nutritional supplement with plenty of Vitamins B and C.

Administer *safe* herbal remedies. Homeopathic remedies are safe to give during pregnancy. Whatever you are doing, whether or not it has been the same for your pet's entire life, you must expect the unexpected during pregnancy. Be careful, always keep a close eye on the mother-to-be for any reactions or stress so you can alter her feeding and supplementation as needed before there is a crisis.

Beneficial and Safe Herbs to Use during Pregnancy

- *Garlic* is wonderfully supportive and nourishing to the growing babies.
- *Yucca Extract* is a safe alternative to steroid use. (See Allergic Reactions.)
- *Ginger Root* and *Peppermint* will control digestive upsets well.
- *Stinging Nettles* is a wonderful antihistamine, a good alternative to *Ephedra*.
- *Burdock Root* can quickly help reverse anemia and strengthen the immune system.
- *Yellow Dock* improves iron assimilation and skin conditions.
- *Bilberry* addresses proper kidney function and supports detoxification.
- *Echinacea Leaf* is a safe immune stimulant and herbal antibiotic.

Beneficial and Safe Homeopathic Remedies to Use during Pregnancy

- *Arsenicum*, *Apis*, and *Nux Vomica* are safe for detoxification, digestive upsets, excessive licking, scratching, and skin eruptions.
- *Nux Vomica* is good for old symptoms which have recurred with pregnancy.
- *Pulsatilla* relieves allergy-related diarrhea during pregnancy, especially if the pet is highly excitable or suffers exhaustion from symptoms that are worse during the day.
- *Alumina* is used for abnormal cravings, small, hard, knotty stool, or difficulty passing stool of any shape or consistency.
- *Sepia* is used for threatened abortion preceded by severe allergies.
- *Phosphorus* helps reduce uterine bleeding.

Ringworm (See Skin Parasites.)

Seizures can be the result of an allergic reaction to chemicals or medications, especially over-the-counter antihistamines. It has been reported that within three to six months of chronic drug use, a pet may develop seizures, which stop as abruptly as they started, when the medication is ceased and detoxification is complete.

Some pets may actually have an allergic reaction to the chronic assault of histamine or adrenaline (as a glandular response to ongoing allergy conditions). This is why it is so important to control these conditions quickly. High levels of *B-Complex* vitamins, *Selenium*, and *Co-Q 10* are appropriate nutritional supplements, if allergies are thought to be involved.

Herbal Remedies for Seizure Disorders

- *Skullcap Herb*, *St. John's Wort*, and *California Poppy* are herbs known for reducing and possibly eliminating seizure activity.
- *Calendula Flowers* rebalances hormones that can stimulate seizures.
- *Chamomile Flowers*, *Valerian Root*, *Hops*, and *Wild Oats* are relaxants that reduce the severity of the seizure activity and resulting digestive upsets.

Homeopathic Remedies for Seizure Disorders

- *Arsenicum* can reverse seizure activity in many cases.
- *Silica* is good for seizures that occur during sleep.
- *Belladonna* reverses seizure activity that follows nausea, vomiting, or constipation.

Straining to evacuate the bowel (as well as the toxins being absorbed) can trigger seizure episodes, so maintaining proper colon health is vital to treating seizures.

Sinusitis (See Infections, Upper Respiratory Problems.)

Skin and Coat Problems occur frequently with many allergy-related conditions. The skin, the largest eliminatory organ, can manifest many symptoms.

Eczema, Hot Spots, Pimples, Cysts, Fatty Tumors, and Warts These skin problems can be reversed with a combination of herbs including *Red Clover, Stinging Nettle Leaf, Cleavers Herb, Yellow Dock Root, Burdock Root*, and *Yarrow Flowers*. Homeopathically, *Apis* addresses rashes and general irritation, resulting in scratching or rubbing. *Thuja* and/or *Arsenicum* help eliminate warts, cysts, and fatty growths, as does *Calcarea Carb*. *Silica* works well for eliminating growths under the skin, including cysts, abscesses, or ulcers. *Hepar sulph* is indicated for weepy, painful areas.

Greasy Coat or Offensive Odors can be addressed through proper grooming followed by an antiseptic rinse. To make an antiseptic rinse cut up one lemon (rind and all). Boil it in one pint of distilled water for five minutes. Then cover and simmer for twenty minutes. Let the lemon sit in the water overnight. Strain in the morning and refrigerate. Add twenty drops of *Golden Seal Extract* or *Grapefruit Extract* if needed for infection control. Homeopathic *Psorinum* is beneficial when the skin has an acrid odor with discharging pustules or hot spots that are slow to heal. *Psorinum* reduces the production of the sebaceous glands, which is associated with a greasy coat and sebaceous cysts.

Dry Coat, Dandruff, Cracked Skin, and Thin Skin should be addressed with herbal formulas containing *Milk Thistle Seed* (for liver toxicity), *Yellow Dock Root* (improves fatty acid metabolism), *Burdock Root* (purifies blood), *Echinacea Root* (antibacterial, anti-ehrlichiosis), *Sarsaparilla Root* (for disorders associated with hormonal balance), and

Oregon Grape Root (aids liver metabolism). *Arsenicum* is a good general homeopathic choice, while *Sepia* works well on irritations (especially cracked toes and feet) that itch badly with no relief from scratching. *Psorinum* can be used for a dirty and dingy coat that is brittle and lackluster. Topical application of *jojoba oil* conditioner can also help temporarily, to reduce dryness, while herbs and nutrients are building up in the body and reversing the underlying imbalance.

Hair Loss, Poor Coat Condition, and Excessive Scratching respond well to *Turmeric Root, Black Catechu, Grindelia Flowers, Licorice Root, Ginkgo Leaf, African Devil's Claw, Yarrow,* and *Lobelia.* Homeopathic *Arsenicum* is best suited for general hair loss. *Sulphur* addresses ringworm or other circular-patch irritations, which are often the cause of scratching and hair loss.

Proper grooming is of paramount importance for stimulating dead coat and skin removal, and supporting circulation. Grooming will bring more nutrients to the skin and coat for tissue repair. A daily brushing followed by a rubdown with a damp terry cloth towel can work wonders. (See Allergic Reactions.)

Skin Parasites can trigger your pet's allergy symptoms. It is prudent to have your pet examined to find out whether a skin parasite is present, so that it may be addressed as one of the underlying problems. Avoid the use of medicated or chemical-based topical pest control treatments, which could possibly depress the immune system and increase your pet's sensitivity to allergic reactions.

Regardless of your findings, the immune system imbalance needs to be addressed. Healthy, non-toxic pets do not encourage infestation. Waste products exuded through the skin will invite and feed fleas and ticks. Yeast, commonly used to ward off fleas and ticks, may become toxic to the liver, increasing instances of infestation. Ear wax and debris also develop, providing a receptive area for bacterial and yeast infections, which attract ear mites.

Common Parasitic Infestations
Associated with Allergy Conditions

- *Demodex Mites* are vicious skin parasites, that burrow down into the epidermis, causing *Demodactic Mange*, which results in a great deal of discomfort and irritation. Scratching and chewing can quickly lead to infection with discharge. Puppies and chronically ill or elderly pets are particularly susceptible to Demodactic Mange, especially those who have recently been vaccinated.

  Puppies are most often first infested by the bitch, who may not show signs of mange but may be infested with mites. These pups become symptomatic after their young immune systems are compromised. Although they may grow out of it as their immune systems mature, puppies can be very debilitated by chronic mange. Though it can be widespread on the body, it is often located on the head and neck, where it causes skin inflammation and spreading patterns of rashes and hair loss.

  Treat daily with a topical solution of twelve drops *Grapefruit Extract*, six drops each of *Tea Tree Oil*, *Golden Seal Root Extract*, and *Pau d'Arco Extract*, two drops of *Yucca Extract*, and three tablespoons fresh squeezed *lemon juice* diluted in two ounces of *Witch Hazel* and four ounces of distilled water. Let mange area air dry and leave it uncovered.

- *Sarcoptes* are a type of mite that causes *Sarcoptic Mange* in weakened or chronically ill pets. Referred to as "scabies," these mites can burrow into human flesh as well in order to lay eggs. It is vital that you treat the whole household if symptoms appear. Symptoms can include itchy rashes localized around the ears, elbows, and hocks. Scratching can be intense, so *Yucca Extract* should be given orally to reduce inflammation. (See Allergic Reactions.) For a topical solution, see the advice given for *Demodex Mites*.

- *Ear Mites, or Otodectes*, are tiny, white spider-like pests. They are practically impossible to see with the naked eye. They leave a trail of digested blood and debris in the ear, which resembles finely ground pepper and results in a gritty discharge. To dissolve a suspected infestation that is not creating severe pain or bleeding, warm up two tablespoons of *garlic-flavored cooking oil*, to discourage bacterial growth—or use soybean oil and add a capsule of garlic extract—with six drops each of *Golden Seal* and *Mullein Extract*, and 200 IUs of Vitamin E. Apply with a dropper, spoon, or cotton ball, dripping it down into the ear. Allow it to set for as long as your pet will tolerate, at least one-half hour, if possible, to suffocate the mites. Finish by massaging the base of the ear to loosen the debris further before flushing the ear out with a cleaning solution. Repeat several times per day until all the mites are removed, usually within a day or two.

- *Fleas and Ticks* can not only create a lot of problems related to skin disorders but also make treating skin allergies impossible if infestation is allowed to continue. They weaken and can infect the animal with more serious disease. *Diatomaceous earth* (tiny, ground-up fossils which dehydrate the pest's outer coating and therefore kill it) can be an effective barrier between your home or yard and the pests. Clean bedding and pet well with a natural insecticide shampoo and follow with a natural dip. Follow all directions carefully. Groom daily to help remove pests, dead skin and coat, and also to make skin treatments easier.

- *Ringworm* is a fungal infection. It can create many of the same symptoms, such as skin inflammation, itching, and hot spots that are associated with allergies. Ringworm looks like a small, circular area with hair loss and irritation. Scratching can lead to bacterial infection. Treat it topically with mange solution or apply *lavender oil* to those areas.

Once you have correctly identified the problem and specifically addressed it, those symptoms that are associated with your pet's allergies may begin to reverse themselves. Seek additional specific herbal or homeopathic support when needed.

Red Clover Blossoms, Stinging Nettle Leaf, Cleavers Herb, Yellow Dock Root, Burdock Root, Yarrow Flowers, Plantain Leaf and Corm, Licorice Root, and *Prickly Ash Bark* purify the blood and drain excess lymphatic fluids. They are indicated for skin disorders such as mange.

Spilanthes Leaf and Root, Grape Root, Juniper Berry, Usnea Lichen, and *Myrrh Gum* can be effectively used together to reverse ringworm, as can *Sarsaparilla.* These herbs can be used topically and internally. (See Ear Problems, Immune System Disorders, Infection, Skin and Coat Problems.)

Stomach Problems (See Digestive Disorders.)

Ticks (See Skin Parasites.)

Thyroid Problems can be very common in animals that exhibit allergic reactions, especially in chronic skin conditions or weight problems. Often, thyroid problems can be caused by previous cycles of steroid medications, the drugs commonly used to suppress allergy-related symptoms.

Raw glandulars with thyroid, and supportive glandulars such as adrenal and pituitary glands, plus proper nutrition, can often reverse thyroid weakness and rebalance function. *Yucca,* in the standardized extract form, seems to help the thyroid respond more quickly to nutritional support.

Herbal therapy with *Bladderwrack, Thuja Leaf,* and *Blue Flag Root* is good for goiter and thyroid hypoactivity, while *Bugleweed, Motherwort, Lemon Balm,* and *Melissa* are appropriate for thyroid hyperactivity.

Upper Respiratory Problems can be the most difficult chronic symptom to reverse, since the lung and nasal tissues can be so easily irritated by allergens. Damaged from chronic allergy symptoms such as wheezing and discharge, these tissues become even more sensitive. Daily cleaning of the nostrils with a warm, damp cloth to keep discharge and crusted mucus clear of nasal passages will help facilitate healing. Homeopathic and herbal supplementation can successfully address these symptoms. (See Allergy Reactions, Infections.)

Vaccinations can trigger an allergic reaction and weaken the immune system enough to lower resistance to allergens in general. If you suspect that this is the case, then use homeopathic *Arsenicum* and *Thuja* in frequent daily doses until symptoms show signs of reversal. Symptoms can include lethargy, digestive upsets including loss of appetite, and fever. You may also see a discharge from the anus, the nose, the eyes, or the injection site within twelve hours of the shots.

To use these remedies as a preventive and to lessen the likelihood of a reaction, begin dosing a few days prior to the shots. Avoid giving yearly vaccinations during the seasons your pet is most sensitive, or avoid vaccinations altogether by researching homeopathic nosodes made from the actual diseases, such as parvo or FIP. I have had great success with this type of homeopathic protection.

Vomiting (See Digestive Disorders.)

Warts (See Skin and Coat Problems.)

Weight Problems are not uncommon in pets also struggling with allergy-related symptoms. Improper digestion and assimilation (also at the root of allergies) can interfere with the body's ability to utilize calories properly for energy. The brain is responsible for deciding if the body is being fed enough. If nutrients are not available to the blood through proper assimilation, the brain will think that the body is starving. It then decides to store calories as fat, rather than use them as energy to repair tissue and support the immune system. Pets who suffer great anxiety or debilitation along with their allergies can also have trouble maintaining proper weight, regardless of what they are fed.

Herbs, such as *Chickweed, Safflower Flowers, Burdock Root, Parsley, Licorice Root, Hawthorn Berries, Fennel,* and *Cayenne* work together to melt pounds away naturally and to rebalance the digestive tract for greater assimilation.

Siberian Ginseng, Chinese Schizandra Berry, Damiana Leaf, Kola Nut, Wild Oats, Skullcap, and *Prickly Ash* work synergistically to restore integrity to the adrenal glands and to promote weight gain and maintenance. This herbal combination acts as an adaptogen to counter chronic stress, which may be causing weight loss due to allergic reactions. (See Digestive Disorders.)

How to Be Your Vet's Best Friend

The most important ally you can have, in taking care of your pet, is a trusted veterinarian. You should never think that you can handle each and every health concern on your own. You can however, manage your pet's health care yourself, while making all medically-related decisions using the expertise and guidance of a competent professional. Rely on your veterinarian to explain specific genetic weaknesses and local health concerns so that you can develop a sound preventative program around your pet's individual needs.

Yearly health exams and occasional blood work can help catch an imbalance early before it becomes a health problem. Often an imbalance in the endocrine system, protein assimilation, or blood sugar irregularities can be spotted long before the actual symptoms, such as allergies or organ failure, show themselves. This can make the difference between simply reversing an acute weakness or having a chronic condition develop. Proper diagnosis to verify a specific imbalance can make the difference between addressing the problem head-on and more successfully, or trying a "hit or miss" therapy that can go on for months. Monitoring the body as it responds to the chosen therapy will also help you identify generally what is or isn't working.

Today, there are more holistically-oriented veterinarians who are well versed in the complementary modalities of nutritional therapy, herbs, homeopathy, acupuncture, massage and chiropractic care. Some have even expanded to incorporate esoteric therapies of sound, light and energy healing. In addition, a large number of allopathic (traditionally trained) veterinarians now realize that natural pet care has its place within their traditional, medically-based treatments.

Unfortunately, many of us have had very negative experiences with veterinarians—especially those allopathically trained veterinarians who are unfamiliar with natural care and thus are uncompromising. We may now avoid seeking veterinary support. Possibly, they have spoken to us as if we did not have a clue in our heads about our pet's health care needs, or they have dismissed our attempts to seek a chemical-free lifestyle for our pets. More likely, they simply failed to address past conditions successfully, and we have lost faith in the medical approach.

I am hoping that by giving you a little insight as to what can be successfully accomplished with natural modalities, while encouraging you to join forces with your veterinarian—rather than giving them unchallenged authority over your pet's medical care—will empower you so that you can successfully incorporate proper veterinary care in your pet's holistic lifestyle.

It is vital that you seek a veterinarian who is willing to listen to you, is thorough in their examination and diagnosis, will explain what it is that they recommend and why—but most importantly—will treat you and your pet with respect. If you do not like the way a veterinarian approaches your pet or speaks to you, find another, no matter who recommended them.

It becomes very frustrating for a diagnostician when a pet owner doesn't have the most basic information, and puts the veterinarian (who cares) at a disadvantage—in properly identifying what might be a the bottom of the pet's symptoms. Soon, such veterinarians become jaded and assume that all their clients simply don't have a clue. Who can blame them? Open the lines of communication. Learn more about the choices you make and the recommendations given to you by all concerned parties. You know your pet best and this information will help your companion receive better veterinary care.

By making the necessary changes in your pet's lifestyle and health care before a serious problem or chronic condition develops, you will keep them healthy. Prevention is the best cure! The best defense for an allergic pet is a strong offense. The first step is to get a proper diagnosis from your veterinarian to ensure that you are not dealing with a more serious illness or structural disorder. Whatever the problem, serious or minor, there are many natural protocols you and your veterinarian can successfully follow.

Above all, do not give up prematurely. There are no magic bullets. Remember that the more compromised an animal's health is and the longer they have been suffering, the longer it will take to rebalance the body—but nature holds the key.

With this in mind, I have prepared a ten-point health checklist, which I recommend that you read carefully. Please observe your pets so that you understand what they look like when they are healthy. This will enable you to quickly identify and address any weakness or imbalance when it occurs. Have this information available the next time you visit your veterinarian, as it will help them assess the situation correctly.

Nutrition
- What type of food do you feed? How often do you feed?
- Is it well-balanced? Bring in the label if needed.
- Has your pet's eating habits changed recently?
- Do they seem satisfied or always hungry?
- Has your pet's diet changed recently?

- Has the pet's food become rancid due to age or heat?
- Have you introduced any new supplements, treats, chewable toys, or food ingredients that may be creating the problem?

Digestion

- Does your pet have daily bowel movements? Is flatulence a problem, and when?
- Has the stool odor, volume, color, or consistency changed recently?

Major signs of illness can include vomiting, diarrhea, or constipation for more than twenty-four hours. Pancreatic imbalance (fatty, discolored stool) and parasitic infestations (rice or string-like bodies within the stool) can be quickly diagnosed, thereby making them much easier to reverse, and preventing them from developing into more serious conditions such as diabetes or irritable bowel syndrome.

Urination

- Do you allow free access to a potty area?
- Do you impose set potty times around your own schedule? Has this schedule changed?
- Is your pet refusing to use the same litter or potty area as before?
- Has your pet's normal daily intake of water changed?
- Is the urine now painful, scant, or bloody? Is there a metallic or sweet odor to it?
- Has your pet recently become incontinent?

Skin and Coat Condition

- Has there been changes in sheen or general condition?
- Dry flakes, dull coat, or greasy, with hot spots, pimples?
- Excessive shedding, hair loss, scratching or licking, fur pulling?

Coat and skin condition can give you good general information about your pet's health, particularly about the health of the kidney and liver. Toxic waste will often be eliminated through the skin if these organs are not kept in peak condition.

Ears

- Are pests, such as mites (small dark specs like pepper) present for months prior to the immune system taking a serious dive? Have the ears begun to smell?
- Are symptoms related to allergy seasons or weather changes?

Allergies, yeast, or bacterial infections will often first manifest themselves in the ears. Immersion in water (in pools or lakes) can create swimmer's ear in pets as well. When ears are inflamed or have a waxy discharge, it is often the first sign of immune imbalance or toxicity.

Eyes and Nose

- Have infected eyes quickly become matted and painful?
- Is discharge chronic? Or seasonally-related?

Red, swollen eyes are often a window upon the immune system, especially symptomatic of improper liver function and detoxification. Irritated eyes can create blocked tear ducts, manifesting in nasal discharge and respiratory difficulties. Genetic conditions, such as turned-in lashes, can be addressed early on before they can cause permanent damage and even blindness.

Nervous System, Body, Joints, and Muscles

- Has your pet recently shown signs of confusion, lethargy, or uncontrollable shaking?
- Difficulty drinking or eating? Any rapid weight changes?

- Is there any fever or body odor present?
- Has their gait or movement, especially getting up or down, changed?
- Noticeable pain or limping? Restless sleep or exhaustion?

Respiratory and Cardiac

- Has your pet's breathing changed? Can they play as long as they used to before becoming winded?
- Have they developed a cough or wheezing?
- Has their resting pulse rate or breathing patterns changed?

Emotional and Behavioral

- Has your pet recently become withdrawn, fearful, nervous, or aggressive?
- Have they become more destructive in chewing on themselves, furniture, walls, or suddenly soiling in the house?

There can often be a physical problem behind these behavioral issues, just as stress can lead to health problems. Have you or your family recently gone through divorce, moving, death (even of another pet), or other stressful events? Your pets will surely suffer the increased stress in their environment. Often, they suffer more than humans do in such a change—all they understand is that there's a problem. They cannot reason that it might soon be resolved, nor do they know why the change may have occurred. They just worry about the change in their environment and the fact that you, as the center of their universe, are now different in a negative way.

Environment

- Have you recently sprayed the yard for weeds or applied chemical pest control solutions in the house, yard, or even directly on your pet?

- Is your pet wearing a chemically based flea/tick collar?
- Are there any other poisons, radiator fluid, or toxic plants, such as poinsettias, available to your pet to chew on or ingest in some way?
- Have you installed new floor covering that might be seeping formaldehyde or other toxins that your pet is directly exposed to?
- Has the quality of your pet's drinking water or diet changed?
- Have they been given a new medication or recent vaccination?

All of these can trigger a toxic reaction, weaken the immune system, or cause organ failure. Because ninety percent of health problems today are caused by pets' environment, it is vital that you become aware of what it is exactly that your pet is exposed to or ingesting. Once you can answer these questions honestly, you will become more familiar with your pet's ongoing health and be able to keep your pet in optimum condition. By making the necessary changes in their lifestyle and health care before a serious problem or chronic condition arises, you will be able to keep them healthy, and save money to boot. Prevention is the best cure!

By being able to identify any health or behavioral issues that have changed in your pet, you will help your veterinarian assess the underlying problem quickly. Often, due to guilt, an owner will minimize how long a symptom has been present or how severe the condition has actually become. This will only serve to confuse the veterinarian during the intake exam and possibly lead them to a wrong diagnosis.

It is best to address all changes in your pet's health as quickly as possible, but in the event that you have waited or simply did not notice such changes until they became a serious problem, report these facts honestly so that your veterinarian can take this into account.

Blood in the urine is not a good sign, but it isn't considered as serious when it happens for a day or two due to detoxification, and there is improvement in the animal's overall condition. Blood in the urine for a few days with changes in fluid intake, scant output, or painful urination is serious. If you don't know what factor is associated with the bleeding, it's smarter for the veterinarian to assume that the bleeding has been ongoing, rather than assume, based on erroneous information, that it is less serious.

Also, certain foods, supplements, remedies, or herbs that you have been recently using (especially within the last six to eight weeks), may have created a curative response. Taken at face value, these symptoms may lead the veterinarian to suspect a more serious problem. But once you inform the vet about these changes, she/he may feel more confident to support the curative process, rather than suppress the symptoms with medication or a change in remedies.

Also, when you are better informed, your veterinarian will probably have more confidence in your judgment. Many veterinarians, even holistically oriented ones, will rely on drugs to suppress symptoms easily (one or two pills a day), rather than suggest a holistic protocol (fasting, dietary changes, frequent supplementation, or remedy dosing) because they suspect that the owner will simply not be willing to comply and follow through.

Certainly, it can be difficult to decide when to seek veterinarian care or when to try to support your pet's own curative abilities by yourself. Whenever you are in doubt, do seek professional support, but be sure that the vet is someone who you know is competent, who can be trusted, and who is willing to support you in treating your pet naturally.

It is not as vital that you seek out a holistic or alternative care veterinarian as it is that you find someone who is willing to listen to you, who is thorough in their examination and diagnosis, who will explain what it is that they recommend, and, most importantly, who will treat you and your pet with respect. If you do not like the way a veterinarian approaches your pet or speaks to you, then find another, no matter how well recommended they were.

A Good Veterinarian:

- Allows, even requests, that you be present during the exam.
- Makes your pet feel safe and comfortable by not towering above them.
- Is calm and respectful toward the pet and you.
- Does not move the pet abruptly.
- Speaks to you and your pet in soothing, respectful tones.
- Answers all your questions honestly without being condescending.
- Explains the use of certain medications, including shots, prior to prescribing them.
- Discusses the alternatives available, medical or holistic, explaining the costs of each.
- Avoids unnecessary testing, invasive procedures, and surgeries.
- Gives you a realistic prognosis and explains the stages of disease and treatment.
- Takes a complete history, prior to giving you their opinion.
- Is willing to discuss your views and your desire to treat your pet naturally and cost-effectively.
- Is someone both you and your pet like and trust.

The best way to be your vet's best friend is first to be clear about what you want and who you want to take care of you and your pet. I mention both of you here. Isn't the fact that the veterinarian treats your pet well the main issue? Absolutely not!

You will also be in crisis when your pet is in crisis. You will be fearful of the unknown (dis-ease, death, medical costs), concerned about the pain and suffering your friend (and for many it is their *child*) may be experiencing. Often, you will be just as overwhelmed by the situation as your pet is. Therefore, it is crucial to your pet's well-being that the veterinarian is capable of taking care of your needs and fears. If she or he doesn't do so, confusion and fear will most certainly interfere with your judgment and your ability to follow through with his prescribed care.

Anyone who has come home to discover a sick pet and rushed him to the veterinary clinic will tell you what it felt like. Even though they are clear-headed professionals, when faced with this emergency they let experts make decisions for them. And those decisions are very important. Men or women, it makes no difference, we are all vulnerable at one time or another, and it's very important to have allies. Please try to make your vet an ally. A trusted veterinarian who will support you and your pet can make the difference between life and death.

First, you must find this wonderful human being—a qualified veterinarian who will cater to you and your pet. My recommendation is that you begin by asking your friends whom they like and trust (assuming that your friends are like-minded). You might also ask your breeder, groomer, or trainer. Then make a phone call. Is the veterinarian willing to spend five minutes on the phone to tell you their philosophy? Or can you only speak to a secretary or vet tech? If they won't make an effort now, it's probable that they won't care later. If you are pleased with the way you are treated over the phone, make an appointment for a health check-up in order to feel the veterinarian out and allow your pet to get to know them without the additional pressure of being injured or ill. This is crucial—that you and your pet have the opportunity to trust the veterinarian before crisis hits. It will help the veterinarian as well, since they will have a picture of your pet in good health, and therefore be better able to determine what is out of balance when dis-ease or injury hits.

Don't forget to interview the staff also, and take mental notes of how well they work with each other and the veterinarian. Are they respectful of each other or argumentative? How clean is the clinic? Does it smell or have ground-in dirt? Is there urine or stool left on the floor? Do the trays and sinks look well kept? Always ask to see the kennels where they keep pets overnight and for recovery after surgery. Does the clinic have separate areas for cats and dogs so they don't hassle each other, soft lighting to minimize stress, and a clean environment? Ask if they are willing to use your pet's usual diet if she/he has to remain overnight. At one time or another this will be important to you—you may need to board them overnight or leave them for a procedure—so you had better know up front what is going on back there.

One last consideration: Ask if there is another veterinarian whom you could turn to in an emergency if your regular vet was not available. Knowing you have a back-up plan will come in handy if you are faced with an emergency.

Being your vet's best friend through open, honest communication, and teamwork will help ensure that you are totally prepared to address any preventative or rehabilitative issues regarding your pet's health quickly, efficiently, and successfully. You may only see the veterinarian once a year for a check-up, but in the case of a more serious condition or emergency, you need to know whom you can count on because your best friend is counting on you!

THE CROSSING PRESS POCKET PET SERIES

Arthritis
By Lisa Newman
$6.95 • Paper
ISBN 1-58091-003-3

Natural Dog
By Lisa Newman
$6.95 • Paper
ISBN 1-58091-000-9

Natural Cat
By Lisa Newman
$6.95 • Paper
ISBN 1-58091-001-7

Nutrition
By Lisa Newman
$6.95 • Paper
ISBN 1-58091-004-1

Parasites
By Lisa Newman
$6.95 • Paper
ISBN 1-58091-006-8

Skin & Coat Care
By Lisa Newman
$6.95 • Paper
ISBN 1-58091-008-4

Training without Trauma
By Lisa Newman
$6.95 • Paper
ISBN 1-58091-007-6

To receive a current catalog from The Crossing Press
please call toll-free, 800-777-1048.
www.crossingpress.com